OXFORD MEDICAL PUBLICATIONS

DATA HANDLING
IN EPIDEMIOLOGY

DATA HANDLING
IN EPIDEMIOLOGY

Co-ordinating Editor
W. W. HOLLAND
B.Sc., M.D.

*Professor and Head of Department of
Clinical Epidemiology and Social Medicine,
St. Thomas's Hospital Medical School, London*

LONDON
OXFORD UNIVERSITY PRESS
NEW YORK   TORONTO
1970

Oxford University Press, Ely House, London W.1

GLASGOW NEW YORK TORONTO MELBOURNE WELLINGTON
CAPE TOWN SALISBURY IBADAN NAIROBI DAR ES SALAAM LUSAKA ADDIS ABABA
BOMBAY CALCUTTA MADRAS KARACHI LAHORE DACCA
KUALA LUMPUR SINGAPORE HONG KONG TOKYO

SBN 19 264909 4

*Printed in Great Britain by Richard Clay (The Chaucer Press), Ltd.,
Bungay, Suffolk*

CONTENTS

LIST OF CONTRIBUTORS

P. ARMITAGE, M.A., PH.D. Professor of Medical Statistics, London School of Hygiene and Tropical Medicine, London.

A. E. BENNETT, M.B., B.S., D.I.H. Senior Lecturer, Department of Clinical Epidemiology and Social Medicine, St. Thomas's Hospital Medical School, London.

LESTER BRESLOW, M.D. Professor of Preventive and Social Medicine, School of Medicine, University of California, Los Angeles.

P. C. ELWOOD, M.D., D.P.H., D.C.H. Medical Research Council Epidemiology Unit (South Wales), Cardiff.

M. A. HEASMAN, M.R.C.P.E., D.P.H., F.S.S. Co-director, Research and Intelligence Unit, Scottish Home and Health Department, Edinburgh.

W. W. HOLLAND, B.SC., M.D. Professor and Head of Department of Clinical Epidemiology and Social Medicine, St. Thomas's Hospital Medical School, London.

H. S. KASAP, A.I.S. Lecturer, Department of Clinical Epidemiology and Social Medicine, St. Thomas's Hospital Medical School, London.

D. KODLIN, M.D., M.P.H. Biometrician, Permanente Medical Group, Department of Medical Methods Research, Oakland, California.

NEIL KESSEL, M.A., M.D., F.R.C.P., D.P.M. Professor of Psychiatry, University of Manchester.

LOUIS M. F. MASSÉ, M.D., M.P.H., DR.P.H., DR. ÈS L. Professor and Head of Department of Biostatistics, École Nationale de la Santé Publique, Rennes (35), Brittany.

F. J. MASSEY, PH.D. Professor of Biostatistics and Preventive Medicine, School of Public Health, University of California, Los Angeles.

A. E. MAXWELL, M.A., M.ED., PH.D. Professor of Psychological Statistics, Institute of Psychiatry, London.

D. L. MILLER, M.A., M.D., D.P.H. Deputy Director, Epidemiological Research Laboratory, Public Health Laboratory Service, London.

H. V. MUHSAM, DR. ÈS SC. Professor of Demography and Statistics, The Hebrew University of Jerusalem.

VICENTE NAVARRO, M.D., D.M.S.A., DR.P.H. Assistant Professor, Department of Medical Care and Hospitals, The Johns Hopkins University, Baltimore, Maryland.

ROGER D. PARKER, PH.D. Associate Professor, Department of Medical Care and Hospitals, The Johns Hopkins University, Baltimore, Maryland.

JOHN PEMBERTON, M.D., F.R.C.P., D.P.H. Professor and Head of Department of Social and Preventive Medicine, Queen's University of Belfast.

K. UEMURA, M.SC., M.ENG. Chief Statistician, Health Statistical Methodology, World Health Organization, Geneva.

W. E. WATERS, M.B., B.S., D.I.H. Medical Research Council Epidemiology Unit (South Wales), Cardiff.

ACKNOWLEDGEMENTS

THIS volume is based in part on papers delivered at the Fifth Scientific Meeting of the International Epidemiological Association, Primosten, Yugoslavia. The Association acknowledges support for its educational and scientific activities from the following: the Adolph Foundation, the Commonwealth Fund, the Milbank Memorial Fund, the Rockefeller Foundation, the United States Department of Health, Education and Welfare, and the Wellcome Trust.

The first section of CHAPTER 3, Communicable Disease: Preventive Trials, was written by Dr. D. L. Miller, to whom the author wishes to record his thanks.

The author of CHAPTER 5 gratefully acknowledges the valuable comments and suggestions made by Dr. M. Grais on the content of this chapter.

The programme of studies examined in CHAPTER 9 is supported by the Endowment Fund of St. Thomas's Hospital, the Department of Health and Social Security, and the South-West Metropolitan Regional Hospital Board. The authors wish to thank the Lambeth Borough Council, Dr. A. L. Thrower, Mr. S. G. Nicholas, and all members of the Department of Clinical Epidemiology and Social Medicine, including the medical and social science students, who assisted them in this study. Computer facilities were granted by Imperial College, London.

The work described in CHAPTER 14 was supported by a research grant CH–00158–04 from the United States Public Health Service, through the National Center for Health Services Research and Development.

Finally, Professor W. W. Holland would like to thank his editorial assistant, Miss C. M. Watson, for her help in the preparation of this book.

INTRODUCTION

INTRODUCTION

P. Armitage

EPIDEMIOLOGY, STATISTICS AND COMPUTERS

THIS book is concerned with problems of data handling in large-scale epidemiological studies. It is not a textbook on either statistics or epidemiology. At some future time it will no doubt be possible for a single author to write an authoritative textbook on our present subject, but the Editors believe that at a time of rapid technical change and expansion of research activities a collection of articles by many authors is of particular interest. This multiple authorship has enabled the Editors to call on experts with very varied specialized interests—a point of particular importance in this interdisciplinary field.

Large-scale quantitative studies in epidemiology give rise to a wide variety of problems, which are discussed in this book in chronological order. The first of these occur at the planning stage: the precise purpose of the study must be defined and its design decided in some detail. Considerable thought will be given to the precise nature of the information required and to the best methods of obtaining the relevant data. The latter will then be processed, and this is increasingly being carried out by automatic data processing with a computer. The information received will be subjected to some form of statistical analysis, and finally the results must be interpreted and correctly related to the existing body of knowledge.

In the chapters which follow the reader will detect a recurrent interplay between the three disciplines of computer science and technology, epidemiology, and statistics. The advent of automatic digital computers has already had a tremendous effect on the scale of data analysis in epidemiological studies. It has, moreover, permitted the introduction of forms of analysis which would have been impracticable before, and has set a new standard in reliability; for example, by encouraging extensive data editing. Part V in particular is devoted to data processing, with special emphasis on computer techniques, but in many of the other chapters too the reader will find constant reminders of the impact of the computer.

The other two disciplines mentioned above, epidemiology and statistics, have a much longer history, and perhaps because of their unfettered growth, particularly over the last half-century, they often defy exact definition. It may therefore be useful to devote the remainder of this introductory chapter to remarks on the role of statistics in epidemiological research and the ways in which this role is changing.

From time to time some enthusiast is heard to claim that medical statistics includes epidemiology or vice versa. Certainly the two terms denote branches of study which are ill-defined and overlap. Many of the pioneers of medical statistics—Farr, Greenwood, and Pearl, for example—were concerned greatly with problems which we might now classify as epidemiological. It is still possible for a medical statistician to occupy this central position, but there is an increasing tendency towards specialization, with medically qualified workers forming the main core of epidemiologists and those with a more mathematical background providing the statistical expertise. This seems to me a natural consequence of the penetration of epidemiological methods into more and more branches of medicine, with an increasing use of clinical techniques and, on the other hand, the development of theoretical statistics. Recently, as we have seen, data processing has appeared as a third branch of study which must play its part in epidemiological research. Sometimes, expertise in data processing may be acquired to a sufficient extent by either an epidemiologist or a statistician. There will be other occasions, however, when the data processing expert or computer scientist is called in as a full research collaborator in his own right.

As I see it, then, medical statistics and epidemiology overlap in their spheres of influence. Epidemiology, as the study of mass phenomena of disease, uses many tools, of which statistical techniques form one group. Statistics, as the discipline concerned with observations on groups of individuals, is applied to many branches of science and medicine, of which epidemiology is one. There is much to be gained by a sympathetic collaboration between practitioners in the two fields. The medically qualified epidemiologist can inform himself about the basic ideas and techniques of statistics without delving very much below the mathematical surface. The mysteries of Banach space may remain forever hidden, but then so they do from most statisticians. Conversely, as Hill (1953) remarked, 'The biostatistician must . . . acquire a taste for lying down with the epidemiologist'; he hastens to add '(I speak in fables)'.

THE SCOPE OF STATISTICS

Statistics is a many-tentacled study. It creeps into the field of data processing, introducing topics like design of questionnaires and the handling of large-scale survey data; into demography, with techniques for handling death-rates; into mathematics, with many of the more abstract developments in theoretical statistics; and, as we have seen, it creeps into epidemiology. Ideally, a statistician engaged in epidemiological research or in advising epidemiologists should develop his own set of tentacles so that he can keep some sort of grip on developments in all these directions. In practice, however, he is unlikely to reach the farthest limits in any one direction.

To illustrate this variety of approach I shall briefly discuss three different types of statistical work, namely, descriptive statistics, inferential methods, and mathematical models, with some examples of the way in which they can be of use in epidemiological research. Finally, I shall refer to some problems which, in particular, arise in the analysis of survey data. The remarks made can be regarded as an introduction to the more specialized sections on statistical analysis in Part VI.

DESCRIPTIVE STATISTICS

The term 'descriptive statistics' is used to denote the procedures of summary and presentation which at one time constituted almost the whole body of known statistical techniques. A great deal of vital statistics falls under this heading, as does the tabulation of data from surveys and other large studies. The epidemiologist must rely heavily on these methods. Some excellent illustrations of the value of descriptive statistics in developing an epidemiological argument are contained in a recent paper by Speizer, Doll, and Heaf (1968) on the recent increase in mortality from asthma. They examine time trends in the numbers of deaths attributed to asthma, giving both crude and age-specific death-rates. Marked increases were observed in England and Wales between 1960 and 1965, particularly at the ages of 10–14 years. Smaller increases took place in other countries. A study of other respiratory diseases shows no compensatory reductions which might be caused by changes in diagnostic criteria. Morbidity data show no increase in prevalence, and it is concluded that the case fatality has risen. Data on changes in the various environmental hazards and methods of treatment are then examined, with the pressurized inhalant emerging as a likely factor. The limitation, as well as the value, of this sort of approach is well brought out by the authors' comment: 'The closeness of the correlation justifies inquiry into the possible harmful effect of the preparations, but a temporal correlation of this sort, taken by itself, is a poor basis for drawing conclusions about cause and effect.' Further evidence, still of a circumstantial nature, is provided by a retrospective study of the use of drugs preceding death from asthma (Speizer et al., 1968).

INFERENTIAL METHODS

When data have been summarized and presented descriptively the conclusions to be drawn from them may be clear enough. This is likely to be so only when the tabulations are reasonably simple, involving associations between, say, not more than two variables at a time or subdivisions of the data into merely two-way classifications. With more complex data some formal assistance is almost invariably needed before reliable inferences can be drawn. There are two main problems: how to sort out the separate effects of many variables which are interrelated in a complicated way, and how to allow for the effect of random error. This is the sort of situation in which the main body of statistical methodology, with its formal methods of statistical inference, comes into its own.

The various types of epidemiological inquiry may draw on different branches of statistical methodology, and occasionally give rise to their own special problems of analysis. There is, for example, a well-established body of statistical methods for the design and analysis of population surveys which epidemiologists should find relevant in conducting prevalence studies. The special problems of surveys designed to detect associations, such as case control or cohort studies of aetiological hypotheses, have been less thoroughly studied. I shall refer to some of these problems later.

Another important branch of inferential statistics is the theory of experimental design. The basic principles of randomization and blocking have had an important influence on the conduct of trials in clinical and preventive medicine. They have had less effect on epidemiology which must, perforce, proceed mainly by non-experimental means. Experimentation plays, of course, an important part in laboratory studies of the epidemiology of infectious diseases, and we may expect it in future to take a more prominent place in field studies. I am thinking here of field trials to test the efficacy of preventive measures in chronic disease, of measures for population control or for health education, and of alternative proposals for the organization of health services. In all these fields the effectiveness of a particular measure might be strongly supported by *a priori* reasoning or by inferences from uncontrolled data; its crucial test can come only from a controlled study in which the new measure is compared with a simultaneous control on a basis of random allocation.

Many epidemiological data are highly multivariate, that is, many variables are measured or observed in the same individual. The analysis of such data gives rise to special problems. For the theoretical background of multivariate analysis is complicated, and many of its results are of doubtful relevance to the sorts of data encountered and the problems posed in epidemiology. Maxwell discusses this subject in more detail in CHAPTER 12.

Recently, statistical methods have been devised for two examples of detection work on diseases whose epidemiology is incompletely understood. One concerns the effect of variations in meteorological factors on the incidence of an infectious disease like poliomyelitis. Such factors, like the disease itself, tend to exhibit cyclical fluctuations throughout a year, so we must be careful that any correlations we find between weather and disease are not due purely to their having a similar pattern of annual fluctuation. An interesting account of the statistical approach to this problem and of some of the results of recent studies is given by Spicer (1967). Secondly, there has been a good deal of interest recently in whether cases of a particular disease, say leukaemia, tend to occur more often in clusters than would be expected to happen purely by chance. Clustering, if present, may have various possible causes. One possibility is an infectious element in the aetiology of the disease. Another is the existence of environmental factors which affect the risk of incurring it. The clustering here must be thought of as being in space and time simultaneously. Clustering in space alone is of no particular interest: people live in geographical clusters and must be expected to die in geographical clusters. Clustering in time alone is almost as unremarkable: we know that the incidence of many diseases changes with time. The data become interesting, however, if the cases which occur close together in time also tend to occur relatively close in space. Various statistical techniques have been proposed (Knox, 1964; Ederer, Myers, and Mantel, 1964; David and Barton, 1966) and have been applied to different sets of data (Mustacchi, David, and Fix, 1967; Lock and Merrington, 1967; Pike, Williams, and Wright, 1967).

MATHEMATICAL MODELS

The statistical techniques discussed in the previous section rely on some sort of mathematical formulation of the way data behave—the nature of the random variation, for instance, or the way in which one variable is affected, on the average, by changing another variable or by moving from one subgroup of the data to another. Such a description is called a 'mathematical model'. The models used in the main body of statistical methodology are relatively simple. For instance, in considering the design and analysis of experiments it is often assumed that the treatments behave in what is known as an additive way; that is, that the effect of using one treatment rather than another is to change the response that would be obtained by adding or subtracting a constant quantity. Another common assumption, often incorporated in the model for the analysis of data, is that a random variable is normally distributed. Assumptions like these are recognized as not being exactly true, but the models are regarded as providing an adequate description of the variation of the data. Their relative simplicity makes them easy to handle mathematically and they have proved to be powerful all-purpose tools.

In some situations, however, these all-purpose models are clearly inadequate. This is particularly true where a complex process is developing in time. For an adequate description of an epidemic, of the scheduling of patients through an X-ray department, or of the movement of psychiatric patients to and from various forms of medical care, we need a model much

B

more complex than that needed for, say, a clinical trial to compare two analgesics. The structure of the model should depend strongly on a knowledge of the mechanisms underlying the process. In a model for malaria epidemiology, for example, one should incorporate reasonably accurate mathematical descriptions of the biting habits of mosquitoes, their survival times, the lengths of the incubation cycles of the parasite in mosquito and man, and so on. Some models will be deterministic, in that the relations between the various variables are given precise form, allowing in no way for the play of chance; others are at least partly 'stochastic' or random, since random variation of some form is allowed to enter the picture. Some interesting examples of model building in medicine are given by Bailey (1967). In Part VI Kodlin [CHAPTER 13] describes some models for survivorship data, while Muhsam [CHAPTER 11] discusses the subject more generally.

ANALYSIS OF SURVEY DATA

I return finally to the epidemiological survey, a field in which one might have expected the problems of theoretical statistics, as distinct from data processing, to be fully worked out. Three groups of problems are mentioned, many of them unsolved, which are probably going to need further study. All of them have become particularly pressing with the advent of computer analysis of survey data.

The first group of problems concerns the methods for examining simultaneously the effects of a number of factors. A familiar example is that of making adjustments for age and sex before comparing prevalence rates in different groups of individuals. It has been traditional to use methods of standardization closely related to those used in vital statistics. However, different methods may give different results; some are convenient for testing a hypothesis that no real difference exists between groups, but are less effective for estimating how big a difference there really is—sampling errors are often awkward to calculate. A rather different approach is to explore the simultaneous effect of the standardizing variables and of the classification into groups, by multiple regression. When the response variable is a proportion, such as a prevalence rate, some sort of transformation is required; the logit transform may well prove to be the most useful (Armitage, 1967a). The logit method has been used in prognostic studies (Armitage, 1967b; Walker and Duncan, 1967; Armitage, Copas, and McPherson, 1969), where its close relationship to discriminant analysis has been noted (Radhakrishna, 1964; Truett, Cornfield, and Kannel, 1967).

The second group of problems is concerned with what Selvin and Stuart (1966) call 'data-dredging': the testing of hypotheses suggested by the data. There is, after all, an infinite number of questions which one could pose about any set of data. If one selects mainly those questions to which the data happen to provide interesting answers, the latter will frequently be misleading. Many of the differences and associations will have arisen by chance and nominal probability levels will be meaningless. For example, in studying differences between subgroups of data there is a temptation to lay too much emphasis on the most extreme contrast that happens to arise. This situation has received a good deal of attention under the heading 'multiple comparisons'. A rather different situation arises in an aetiological study in which correlations are being sought between some disease characteristic and a large number of possible aetiological factors. Some of these are likely to be significant purely by chance, and some degree of caution should therefore be displayed. However, there is no body of theory to guide us here comparable to that in the case of multiple comparison. A different problem again arises in the choice of transformations of variables. In regression analysis one often chooses scales of measurement so that, if possible, relationships are linear and various other desirable statistical properties hold. Now, any transformations used will normally be chosen after the data are examined; they are likely to perform rather more favourably on these particular observations than on subsequent sets of data. Similar points arise in prognosis. Systems for predicting success or failure are likely to work better on the data from which they are derived than on subsequent data (Armitage, 1967b).

It would be quite wrong to discourage imaginative explorations of data. Nevertheless, it seems difficult to allow satisfactorily for selective effects of the type of data I have discussed. Ideally, hypotheses suggested by data should be tested on independent sets of data, but this may be asking too much. Another device is that of the reserved subsample in which a proportion of the observations is reserved for testing hypotheses suggested by the analysis of the remainder. There is room for research into the optimal size of such a subsample. If it is too small the crucial test will be unduly insensitive; if too many observations are reserved, however, the initial analysis may be greatly weakened.

The third and final point is the treatment of outlying observations. One of the important contributions of the computer is the editing of data before analysis to remove gross errors and inconsistencies. There is an obvious danger in thus removing some of the more flamboyant manifestations of variability, but I think few people would agree that data editing should *never* be done. The question immediately arises: how gross is a gross error? Where do we draw the line between acceptable eccentricity and intolerable nonsense? Most field workers would probably rely on intuition and experience. However, there is a good deal of statistical theory about the rejection of outlying observations, from which rigorous rules of rejection have been developed. Anscombe (1960), for instance, thinks of a rejection rule as analogous to an insurance policy. In adopting a rule one pays a premium which in this case is a slight loss of efficiency due to the occasional rejection of valid observations. In return one receives very good protection against the inclusion of gross errors. It would, I think, be useful to consider such procedures in the context of epidemiological survey data. Modifications would no doubt be necessary, for instance by allowing for non-normal distributions, but there may be some merit in adopting procedures with known properties rather than relying purely on intuition.

My own interest in statistical analysis has perhaps steered this introductory chapter further in one direction than is proper in a symposium of this kind. I return, therefore, to the point of departure. The handling of data from large-scale epidemiological investigations is a collaborative activity. If it presents difficulties it also presents opportunities. The following pages show us how these opportunities are being seized.

REFERENCES

ANSCOMBE, F. J. (1960) Rejection of outliers, *Technometrics*, **2**, 123.

ARMITAGE, P. (1967a) Discussion on 'Models for use in investigating the risk of mortality from lung cancer and bronchitis' by Buck, S. F., and Wicken, A. J., *Appl. Statist.*, **16**, 185 (p. 203).

ARMITAGE, P. (1967b) Recenti sviluppi nel'analisi statistica di esperimenti clinici controllati e di inchieste mediche, *Applicazione bio-mediche del calcolo elettronico*, **2**, 123.

ARMITAGE, P., COPAS, J., and McPHERSON, C. K. (1969) Statistical studies of prognosis in advanced breast cancer, *J. chron. Dis.*, **22**, 343.

BAILEY, N. T. J. (1967) *The Mathematical Approach to Biology and Medicine*, New York.

DAVID, F. N., and BARTON, D. E. (1966) Two space-time interaction tests for epidemicity, *Brit. J. prev. soc. Med.*, **20**, 44.

EDERER, F., MYERS, M. H., and MANTEL, N. (1964) A statistical problem in space and time: do leukaemia cases come in clusters?, *Biometrics*, **20**, 626.

HILL, A. B. (1953) Observation and experiment, *New Engl. J. Med.*, **248**, 995.

KNOX, E. G. (1964) Epidemiology of childhood leukaemia in Northumberland and Durham, *Brit. J. prev. soc. Med.*, **18**, 17.

LOCK, S. P., and MERRINGTON, M. (1967) Leukaemia in Lewisham (1957–61), *Brit. med. J.*, **3**, 759.

MUSTACCHI, P., DAVID, F. N., and FIX, E. (1967) Three tests for space-time interaction: a comparative evaluation, *Proc. Fifth Berkeley Symp. Math. Statist. Probab.*, **4**, 229.

PIKE, M. C., WILLIAMS, E. H., and WRIGHT, B. (1967) Burkitt's tumour in the West Nile District of Uganda 1961–5, *Brit. med. J.*, **2**, 395.

RADHAKRISHNA, S. (1964) Discrimination analysis in medicine, *Statistician*, **14**, 147.

SELVIN, H. C., and STUART, A. (1966) Data-dredging procedures in survey analysis, *Amer. Statistician*, **20**(3), 20.

SPEIZER, F. E., DOLL, R., and HEAF, P. (1968) Observations on recent increase in mortality from asthma, *Brit. med. J.*, **1**, 335.

SPEIZER, F. E., DOLL, R., HEAF, P., and STRANG, L. B. (1968) Investigations into use of drugs preceding death from asthma, *Brit. med. J.*, **1**, 339.

SPICER, C. C. (1967) Some empirical studies in epidemiology, *Proc. Fifth Berkeley Symp. Math. Statist. Probab.*, **4**, 207.

TRUETT, J., CORNFIELD, J., and KANNEL, W. (1967) A multivariate analysis of the risk of coronary heart disease in Framingham, *J. chron. Dis.*, **20**, 511.

WALKER, S. H., and DUNCAN, D. B. (1967) Estimation of the probability of an event as a function of several independent variables, *Biometrika*, **54**, 167.

PART I

ASKING THE QUESTIONS

INTRODUCTION

THE basic questions which all those who are concerned with the problems of disease must ask are: 'What has gone wrong?'; 'How can it be put right?'; 'How can it be prevented in future?'

Epidemiology, like pathology or clinical medicine, is one way of studying disease which offers techniques for the investigation of these basic questions. To the pathologist disease is something that happens to cells and organs, to the clinician something that happens to his patient, and to the epidemiologist something that happens to populations. These different concepts cause the investigator concerned to put different questions, and in turn to use different methods of investigation. In the following three chapters we discuss the type of question the epidemiologist asks. The introduction of methods of handling much larger quantities of data than was previously possible, by using the digital computer, has greatly increased the number and complexity of the questions that can now be asked and answered.

The first assumption on which epidemiology rests is that diseases, accidents, and congenital defects are not randomly distributed in the community; many of the questions the epidemiologist investigates can therefore be expressed in the general form: 'What are the reasons for the non-random distribution of a given disease?' In other words, 'Why do some people get it and some not?' To answer this question the epidemiologist logically begins by describing the quantitative distribution of disease in population groups, and seeks to relate his observations to various factors—suspected agents, environmental conditions and host susceptibility—that might influence the distribution. The results may enable him to formulate and test hypotheses about the causation of disease. The second assumption is that the incidence of disease can be modified by intervening in the relationship between man and his environment, which is implicit in the concept of disease prevention. This leads to the questions, 'How can we influence the relationship to man's advantage?' and, 'What is the effectiveness of various preventive measures?'

Epidemiological studies can conveniently be considered under three headings: communicable disease, non-communicable disease, and medical care.

1

COMMUNICABLE DISEASE

D. L. MILLER

THERE are three primary questions concerning the epidemiology of communicable disease: 'What is the agent causing the disease?'; 'How does it reach one host from another?'; and 'What determines whether or not it will cause illness?' From these basic questions flow a series of subsidiary ones concerning the properties of the agent that determine its pathogenicity, the circumstances that favour its transmission, and the factors that affect the relationship between the agent and the host, particularly host immunity. The framing of these questions is almost entirely dependent on an understanding of modern developments in microbiology and immunology, and in epidemiological and statistical techniques for obtaining and handling data. The epidemiologist who wishes to ask sensible questions about communicable disease epidemiology must therefore be familiar with these advances.

MODERN DEVELOPMENTS

With the development of techniques for the culture of bacteria and, more recently, of viruses, it was possible, for the first time, to study diseases defined by reference to the causative organism instead of only on clinical or epidemiological grounds, and to investigate the biological properties of agents that influenced their pathogenicity and mode of spread. It became possible also to inquire into sources of infection in man and in animals, to trace paths of spread and to investigate the importance of environmental contamination and the influence of environmental conditions on the spread of infection. The simple identification of the causative organism, however, is often inadequate to answer such questions. The isolation of *Staphylococcus aureus* from the nose of a surgeon or of *Salmonella typhi* from the faeces of a food handler is insufficient evidence to incriminate that person as the source of associated cases of infection with one of these organisms. The techniques of serological and phage-typing and other methods of 'finger-printing' bacteria of the same species have given added precision to epidemiological inquiries of this kind. With their aid far more sophisticated questions about the sources and paths of spread of infection can be asked.

Equally significant have been advances in immunology. The introduction of the concept of specific immunity and the elaboration of techniques for its measurement provoked inquiry into how antibodies were related to resistance to infection and how the host's resistance to illness could be artificially enhanced. So the search for effective vaccines began. This represented a fundamental shift in the nature of the question being asked about prevention. Formerly the emphasis had been laid on methods of protecting healthy populations from infected persons; the usual solution was to isolate the sick, or otherwise cut the paths of spread. With the discovery of means for giving the individual protection, steps were taken to prevent illness from attacking those who were at present healthy. Nowadays, vaccines have become the principal means of combating many infections. This in turn has led to a series of new questions concerning their protective value, their optimum deployment in preventive programmes, and their continuing safety and efficacy.

The nature of questions that can be asked depends on the availability of suitable techniques for answering them. The techniques used in the routine diagnostic laboratory for the isolation of micro-organisms, particularly for virus isolations, tend to be laborious and not well suited to epidemiological inquiries. The clinician may need to know a good deal about the properties of infecting organisms. The epidemiologist requires tests that are simple to use in the examination of large population groups and capable of discriminating with accuracy between infected and non-infected, or between immune and non-immune, persons. Too little attention has been paid by microbiologists to these needs. Some new laboratory techniques, however, seem likely to prove increasingly useful tools for epidemiological studies. For example, immunofluorescence is becoming firmly established as a means of rapid diagnosis of a wide variety of infections (McEntegart, 1969; Fraser, 1969) and could be valuable in mass screening surveys. Likewise, the development of automated serological tests will provide the facilities required for routine monitoring of the prevalence of specific infections and of immunity in large population groups (Taylor, 1969). Mechanization in the bacteriological laboratory will also assist epidemiological survey work (Williams and Trotman, 1969). The practical importance of laboratory techniques developed specifically for field survey use was shown in a recent study of health problems in village communities in Peru (Buck, Sasaki, and Anderson, 1968).

The collection of reliable mortality statistics is rapidly becoming a routine practice in all parts of the world, and the reporting of cases of serious disease such as smallpox has also greatly improved. These records, which are discussed by Uemura in CHAPTER 5, are of the utmost importance when planning control measures and for assessing their effectiveness. In countries where the recording of deaths and the compulsory notification of certain communicable diseases has been an established routine for many years, new and better sources of morbidity data are now being developed. The Royal College of General Practitioners, for instance, receives routine records of total sickness treated by family doctors in selected practices throughout the United Kingdom (College of General Practitioners, 1963), and in the United States the National Health Survey continuously records sickness prevalence in samples of the population (United States National Center for Health Statistics, 1963). These and other similar schemes provide valuable surveillance data on a wide range of diseases, and enable questions to be asked about disease incidence in a variety of different population groups.

DEFINING THE PROBLEMS

How does the modern epidemiologist set about deciding what questions to ask about communicable disease? It is convenient to divide them into three categories: those relating to the properties of the agent that affect its pathogenicity and mode of spread; those about environmental conditions that assist spread; and those that concern the host's ability to resist infection and the illnesses that may result.

Questions about the Agent

A wide range of biological properties of microbes, involving their nutritional and environmental requirements for survival, growth, and multiplication, influences their pathogenicity and spread. Some, like malaria parasites or the arboviruses, have a life-cycle that requires the presence of an intermediate host; some are better able to withstand or adapt to adverse environmental conditions than others; microbes also vary in their invasiveness and virulence, depending on whether or not they produce toxins or enzymes, and on the site which they infect. Thus, one of the epidemiologist's first questions must be how these properties affect the epidemiological behaviour of different organisms, and the diseases which they cause. For instance, it is important to know that the typhoid bacillus, usually an aerobic organism, can survive and multiply under anaerobic conditions. This lesson was well illustrated by the 1963 outbreak of typhoid in Aberdeen which was probably caused by canned corned beef that had been contaminated by the use of unchlorinated river water for cooling sterilized cans (Scottish Home and Health Department, 1964).

Some microbes are liable to vary in pathogenicity and virulence as a result of changes in antigenic composition. The question is how these changes arise and whether they can be predicted. This problem is particularly familiar to those concerned with influenza, where the difficulty in predicting the behaviour of epidemics and of producing satisfactory vaccines stems largely from the antigenic instability of the virus. Another recently recognized problem which has many important and menacing implications is the capacity for genetic transfer of drug resistance, between organisms both of the same and of different species (Anderson, 1968).

New agents, mostly viruses, are still being discovered in profusion, some associated with acute illness, others in apparently healthy persons. It seems probable, too, that some chronic diseases which hitherto have not usually been regarded as communicable, such as neoplasms and multiple sclerosis, may be caused by living agents. These discoveries raise many complex questions for the epidemiologist. The isolation of an organism, even in association with illness, is not proof that it causes disease. It has become clear, too, that many agents may cause similar clinical illnesses and, conversely, that infection with one agent may be manifested in a variety of ways. Thus, establishing the role of new agents as causes of disease, and other aspects of their epidemiology, requires much careful and systematic study.

Questions about the Environment

Environmental circumstances can affect the incidence of communicable disease either through their influence on the survival and chances of transmission of the agent, or on the resistance of the host. Questions about the environment should be directed, therefore, to such matters as mapping the location of reservoirs of infection, investigating the relation of the life-cycle of the agent to climatic conditions, studying the kind of environmental conditions that favour the spread of infection, and the circumstances that can reduce host resistance. In the past, appreciation of the ways in which poor environmental conditions can affect the distribution of disease and consequent improvements in environmental hygiene have led to some of the most dramatic advances in preventive medicine. Attention to environmental hazards is still important and their removal rewarding—particularly in foodborne diseases (Hobbs, 1968). However, the influence of environment is often complex and presents many unresolved problems: for example, the way in which meteorological conditions affect the incidence of acute respiratory disease, particularly influenza, is still uncertain; moreover, there is a large new area for concern and investigation in the health effects of population migration and rapid urbanization in developing countries. So far as the host is concerned, poor housing, atmospheric pollution, occupational hazards, and a variety of other conditions imposed by cultural, social, and economic patterns of life—all may reduce resistance to infection.

Questions about the Host

Man responds to infection in a variety of ways—he may resist colonization by the microbe entirely, or he may become infected, with or without becoming ill. Questions about what determines this response are of great importance to the epidemiologist, because in the answers lie clues which may enable him to anticipate the course of epidemics and to suggest means of prevention. The questions may be divided into those concerning the immunity of the community as a whole—herd immunity—and those related to the immunity of individuals.

Herd immunity influences the spread, or lack of spread, of a disease which is transmitted from man to man. If the proportion of persons in a community who are immune is high, the agent may not be able to reach susceptible persons often enough to sustain a chain of infection. The proportion of immune persons required to inhibit spread varies with the number of potential sources of infection (i.e. persons shedding the agent), the closeness and frequency of contact between individuals (crowding), and the ease with which the agent spreads. Genetic predisposition also affects population immunity. When, on the one hand, an infection is introduced into a community for the first time, not only is the attack rate likely to be high, but illnesses may be exceptionally severe (Christensen *et al.*, 1952; Adels and Gajdusek, 1963). Where, on the other hand, a disease has been endemic over many generations, natural selection may lead to the survival of a resistant population (Wilson, 1962).

Questions about the immunity of the individual need to consider both non-specific and specific immunity. Non-specific resistance differs with age and sex for physiological reasons, and between races and families, partly, perhaps, for genetic reasons but also, probably, because they are exposed to different environmental conditions, and dietary and social customs. Other factors that influence non-specific immunity, include the state of nutrition, trauma, fatigue, and other disease. Population surveys of specific immunity, measured in terms of serum antibodies, may give much useful information about the prevalence of infection, particularly of otherwise inapparent infection, as well as other data of clinical and epidemiological value (Evans, 1967). But little is known about the way in which amounts of serum antibody are related to past infection and future susceptibility to illness. This question has considerable practical importance in planning immunization and predicting the likely course of epidemics. The results of skin sensitivity tests, such as the tuberculin reaction, are sometimes useful for assessing immunity, and they, too, have been used in surveys of disease prevalence, but their interpretation is often difficult. The role of local antibodies in the cells of the respiratory and gastro-intestinal mucosa in protection against disease is an interesting question that deserves further study. There is no doubt, for instance, of the importance of the 'gut immunity' that results from administration of live virus polio vaccine (Henry *et al.*, 1966).

Agent, Host, and Environment Relations

Questions about the agent, the host, and the environment, although they have been considered separately, are in practice closely interrelated in a dynamic fashion. We cannot simply ask how each factor independently influences the incidence of disease, but require a set of subsidiary questions about how the effect of one is conditioned by the current status of the others. This is an aspect of the epidemiology of communicable disease which has been studied too little. Infection with potentially pathogenic organisms does not always result in disease and, with some infections, illness is the exception rather than the rule. It is important, therefore, to ask what it is that disturbs the balance in the host-parasite relationship. Only by understanding the answers to this question may we make further intelligent and relevant inquiries into methods of maintaining the balance in favour of the host—in other words methods of controlling disease.

PROBLEMS OF CONTROL

The balance between agent, host, and environment may be altered in favour of the host in one of a number of ways—by destroying the agent or its reservoir, by interrupting its paths of spread, or by increasing host resistance. For each disease the question is, 'Which of these approaches is the most efficient, practical, and economic?'

Reservoirs of Infection

The reservoirs of infection may lie in human cases—apparent and inapparent—or carriers, or in animals or insect vectors. The questions are 'Which?', and 'Can they be easily identified and eliminated?' Much confusion and difficulty may arise from failure to recognize the importance of inapparent human infections, for example of polio or salmonella infection, for this can radically alter the epidemiological picture. The detection of such cases and of carriers may not be easy, particularly if, as with typhoid carriers, excretion of the organism is intermittent. It must also be remembered that the danger from an infected person depends on his ability to disperse organisms and the opportunity to do so; this may vary. For example, carriers of staphylococci do not all disperse the organism to the same extent (Ridley, 1959), and carriers of typhoid are harmless unless they handle food or their excreta are allowed to pollute food or water supplies. Where human cases or carriers are the main or only reservoir of infection, as in smallpox, polio, and diphtheria, immunization is an effective means of reducing the pool of infection. Where the reservoir of infection is in animals or insect vectors the remedy lies either in destroying the animals or insects concerned or in eradicating infection from among them. The energetic application of this approach has been successful in controlling such diseases as malaria, rabies, and bovine tuberculosis. Some infections, such as influenza, affect both man and animals, but whether animals act as the primary reservoir in which new antigenic variants originate and then spread to man is uncertain (Tumova, Svandova, and Stumpa, 1968).

Transmission of Infection

When inquiring into the transmission of infection it is important to ask not only how diseases *may be* spread, but how they are most often *actually* spread. This depends on how the agent leaves its first host, how well it can survive in transit, how it enters the new host and the amount of the dose required to infect. In some diseases, such as those spread by insect vectors or by direct personal contact, the mode of transmission is relatively straight-forward and the method of control is correspondingly clear. In others, such as airborne infections and those spread by indirect contact, the mechanics of spread are much more complex and control presents greater problems. Attempts to control the spread of respiratory virus infections by air steriliza-tion, for example, have been unrewarding (Kingston, Lidwell, and Williams, 1962) and alternative approaches may have to be found. Control of cross-infection in surgical wards has also proved an intractable problem and presents a continuing challenge to epidemiologists. The danger of transmission of infection in food and water supplies finds its most dramatic expression in the continuing problems of endemic cholera and typhoid in many of the less developed countries. But even in developed countries food poisoning remains a major problem (Vernon, 1969) due, usually, to lapses in good hygienic practice. With the mass production and distribution of food, such lapses are likely to carry serious consequences when they occur. The food responsible for outbreaks can often be traced with relative ease, but it is much more difficult to discover how foods become contaminated in the first instance and how the cycle of infection is maintained. Salmonella infection is common in livestock and poultry, and the same species of organism may frequently be isolated from other sources such as animal foodstuffs and fertilizers (Report, 1965). But the question of the relative importance of these sources in main-taining infection and in the contamination of food products is unresolved.

The chances of transmission of infection are being increased by the growth of urban living and of population mobility. This is particularly a problem in developing countries, where large numbers of persons with little natural immunity are migrating to towns where the poor environmental conditions are likely to favour the spread of infectious diseases, such as poliomyelitis and tuberculosis. For developed countries, the problem is one of guarding against the introduction of infection from endemic areas, either by travellers or by infected foods and other materials.

Immunization

The host's ability to resist infection may be significantly improved in the long term by general measures, such as improved nutrition, although the benefits are difficult to assess. Occasionally prophylactic antibacterial drugs have a place in controlling infection: for example, penicillin may be useful in the management of outbreaks of streptococcal infection in institutions and in the prevention of wound sepsis. The value of such prophylaxis has been extensively investigated but its proper use is still debated. The usual and generally most satisfactory means of increasing resistance to infection is artificial immunization—either passive prophylaxis with specific antisera or immunoglobulin, or active immunization with vaccines. The value of some antitoxins, notably of tetanus and diphtheria, is undisputed, but the usefulness of immunoglobulin is established in only a few diseases (Miller, 1970). The optimum use of vaccines poses many questions. For the individual, the question is, 'Which diseases does he require protection against in his particular circumstance of life?' This is a matter of weighing the chances of exposure, and the seriousness of the consequences if infection occurs, against the risks of vaccination, which is not without hazards (Wilson, 1967). As long as the chances of contracting a disease are high and the consequences dangerous, even occasionally serious reactions to vaccination may be acceptable, but, if the disease is rare, as in the case of smallpox in most countries, adverse reactions are viewed more critically. It may then be asked whether vaccines should not be used selectively to protect contacts and those at special risk, such as medical personnel and travellers to endemic areas. The duration of immunity is also important. Where the consequences of infection are serious this question is unlikely to be decisive; but for diseases that are usually benign, such as the exanthemata of childhood and respiratory virus diseases, immunity should, for practical purposes, be lifelong. This question has been hotly debated in relation to the use of measles vaccine and will undoubtedly arise with other vaccines as time goes on.

For the community, it may be asked how far vaccination can be expected to control a disease and whether protection of certain groups can be relied on to protect others. By raising the level of herd immunity, it may be possible to reach a point that prevents or limits the spread of infection without the necessity of protecting all individuals. Poliomyelitis has been almost eliminated in many countries in this manner, and the incidence of measles in the United States has been reduced to a very low rate (United States Public Health Service, 1969a). It is of great importance, therefore, to determine the level of herd immunity which must be achieved for any particular infection in order to control it. It may also be asked whether, by concentrating vaccination on those most likely to spread infection, vulnerable groups can be protected. This approach has been adopted with pertussis vaccine in the past and is proposed for rubella vaccine: by immunizing older siblings against pertussis it was hoped indirectly to protect young infants and, similarly, by immunizing school children against rubella it is now hoped to prevent spread to pregnant mothers (United States Public Health Service, 1969b).

There is a tendency to assume that once a vaccine has been developed and its efficacy and safety demonstrated, this is adequate justification for advocating its general and continuing use. This should not be unquestioned. Its value should be judged in relation to other methods of control. It should be asked whether it is justified to divert medical resources from these other methods in order to carry out mass vaccination, for example with BCG, in a situation where the incidence of the disease is declining.

Eradication

One of the most important recent changes in attitude to communicable disease is that, instead of control, the aim, at least for some infections such as yaws, malaria and smallpox (Guthe and Idsoe, 1968; World Health Organization, 1968a and b), has become eradication. Is this possible? Some are optimistic that it is (Andrews and Langmuir, 1963); others are sceptical (MacLeod, 1963). Whether or not this is an attainable objective, epidemiologists will have no doubt that it is a question well worth asking. In diseases which have a single reservoir or mode of transmission which can be attacked and destroyed, such as bovine tuberculosis or malaria, or an agent that is highly susceptible to antimicrobial drugs, like yaws, or where there exists an effective vaccine and man is the only host, as in poliomyelitis or smallpox, eradication probably can be attained. Much success, for example with smallpox (Cockburn, 1966), has already been recorded although progress has not always been easy, particularly with malaria (*Lancet*, 1970). The adaptability of microbes and the practical difficulties of locating and destroying residual reservoirs must not be underestimated. Diseases with a more complex epidemiology, and microbes whose pathogenicity varies, such as streptococci and influenza virus, may never be totally eradicable, although they may eventually be closely controlled. The problems of eradication are likely to be a major preoccupation of epidemiologists for a long time to come.

SURVEILLANCE

The distribution of communicable diseases is liable to continual change due to changes in the behaviour of the agent, environmental circumstances and population immunity. Changes are often insidious, and without surveillance may easily pass unnoticed and unchecked in their earliest stages. Here the question is 'What is currently happening in communicable diseases?' The modern concept of surveillance involves the continuous collection and analysis not only of morbidity and mortality statistics, which is essential, but also of data on all the circumstances that determine the incidence of communicable disease in human populations, such as vector distribution and insecticide susceptibility, bacteriological safety of food and water supplies, vaccination records and population immunity, and—most important—the regular dissemination of information to those with responsibilities for disease control (World Health Organization, 1968c).

C

Surveillance serves in the first place to detect outbreaks. In addition, it defines problems requiring planned investigation, provides a scientific basis for advising on control measures and the constitution of vaccines, and assists in planning the best use of medical resources. Continuing surveillance of the efficacy and safety of vaccines is particularly important, as was emphasized by the notorious Cutter incident, in which cases of paralytic polio-myelitis followed administration of incompletely inactivated poliovirus vaccine (Nathanson and Langmuir, 1963). As a result poliomyelitis has been kept under careful surveillance, particularly since the introduction of live virus vaccines, for any evidence of vaccine-induced disease (Henderson *et al.*, 1964; Miller and Galbraith, 1965). Surveillance of all vaccines is now becoming routine.

Responsibility for surveillance is usually vested primarily with local health authorities. But this alone is insufficient: the conditions of modern life—increased travel, population mobility, mass production and distribution of foodstuffs—make provision of well-integrated and comprehensive national and international surveillance increasingly necessary, and in this respect the World Health Organization has taken a strong lead (Raška, 1966; World Health Organization, 1968c).

INVESTIGATION OF OUTBREAKS

Outbreaks of communicable disease can occur with dramatic suddenness and carry serious consequences. The questions then are urgent and doctors and public alike clamour for quick answers. The epidemiologist must be well prepared if he is to handle the situation with equanimity. Each outbreak, even of the same disease, is different and requires managing in its own way; but this is no excuse for unplanned inquiry. The questions that need to be asked must be devised in advance, and the means of organizing investigations established. In particular, there must be arrangements for co-ordination between all concerned—clinicians, laboratory director, and public health workers.

The questions for the epidemiologist are:

'What is the source?',
'How has it or may it spread?',
'Who is affected?',
'How can it be controlled?'

To answer these requires a sound knowledge of the clinical features and epidemiology of the disease in question. First, the incidence of cases in relation to time, place, and persons affected is determined and appropriate clinical and laboratory investigations to establish the cause are carried out. Patients and others concerned in the outbreak are questioned to identify the characteristics and experiences that affected groups of persons have in common. The incidence of illness may then be compared in those who have and have not been exposed to suspected sources of infection and the course of the epidemic charted. In order to establish the mode of infection, possible sources and vehicles of infection are investigated, supported where necessary by laboratory tests. Phage- and serological typing may help to link cases with one another and with the suspected source. From analysis of this kind of information a working hypothesis may usually be formed on which to base further investigations and institute control measures.

THE FUTURE

What are likely to be the most important questions for the future? First, we need to know much more about the nature of the relationship between micro-organisms and man. What are the determinants of the microbe's pathogenicity and of man's susceptibility? As new agents are discovered their epidemiological features will need to be systematically studied. This task has only just begun for the large groups of newly-discovered respiratory viruses and enteroviruses. Epidemiological inquiries may help to establish whether viruses have a role in human oncogenesis and to determine how slow virus and latent virus infections are related to human disease. In addition, the epidemiology of some of the more familiar bacterial causes of diseases, such as streptococci and staphylococci, still poses many questions.

What can be done to increase man's ability to resist infection? Immunization is one way, but it is cumbersome, sometimes hazardous, and not an indefinitely extendible exercise. There may be other, more efficient means of achieving the same objective.

Questions concerning control and eradication of communicable disease are most pressing in the developing countries and must continue to have high priority. But even in developed areas of the world the recrudescence of venereal disease, particularly gonorrhoea, reminds us that problems of control are continuing ones. Changes in social structure and man's own follies may open new routes of infection: the introduction of 'battery' rearing of poultry and animals and the use of antibiotics in animal foodstuffs, for example, have created serious new problems in the epidemiology of salmonellosis and the spread of antibiotic-resistant enterobacteria. Operational research using mathematical models may help in the tailoring of control measures designed to obtain optimum performance in any given set of conditions. This should greatly assist in the conservation of medical resources, which is vitally important, particularly in developing countries where such resources are scarce.

Finally, there is surveillance. Comprehensive surveillance serves to detect what is happening, and to anticipate and forestall what may happen. It not only alerts to danger, but is the basis on which most other questions in communicable disease epidemiology are built.

REFERENCES

ADELS, B. R., and GAJDUSEK, D. C. (1963) Survey of measles patterns in New Guinea, Micronesia and Australia. With a report of new virgin soil epidemics and the demonstration of susceptible primitive populations by serology, *Amer. J. Hyg.*, **77**, 317.

ANDERSON, E. S. (1968) Drug resistance in *Salmonella typhimurium* and its implications, *Brit. med. J.*, **3**, 333.

ANDREWS, J. M., and LANGMUIR, A. D. (1963) The philosophy of disease eradication, *Amer. J. publ. Hlth*, **53**, 1.

BUCK, A. A., SASAKI, T. T., and ANDERSON, R. I. (1968) *Health and Disease in Four Peruvian Villages. Contrast in Epidemiology*, Baltimore, Md.

CHRISTENSEN, P. E., SCHMIDT, H., JENSEN, O., BANG, H. O., ANDERSON, V., and JORDAL, B. (1952) An epidemic of measles in southern Greenland, 1951. Measles in virgin soil. I, *Acta med. scand.*, **144**, 313.

COCKBURN, W. C. (1966) Progress in international smallpox eradication, *Amer. J. publ. Hlth*, **56**, 1628.

COLLEGE OF GENERAL PRACTITIONERS (1963) The records and statistical unit, *J. Coll. gen. Practit.*, **6**, 195.

EVANS, A. S. (1967) Serological surveys. The role of the WHO reference serum bank, *Chron. Wld Hlth Org.*, **21**, 185.

FRASER, K. B. (1969) Immunological tracing: viruses and rickettsiae, in *Fluorescent Protein Tracing*, 3rd ed., ed. Nairn, R. C., Edinburgh (Chapter 8).

GUTHE, T., and IDSOE, O. (1968) The rise and fall of the treponematoses. II. Endemic treponematoses of childhood, *Brit. J. vener. Dis.*, **44**, 35.

HENDERSON, D. A., WITTE, J. J., MORRIS, L., and LANGMUIR, A. D. (1964) Paralytic disease associated with oral polio vaccines, *J. Amer. med. Ass.*, **190**, 41.

HENRY, J. L., JAIKARAN, E. S., DAVIES, J. R., TOMLINSON, A. J. H., MASON, P. J., BARNES, J. M., and BEALE, A. J. (1966) A study of polio vaccination in infancy: excretion following challenge with live virus by children given killed or living polio vaccine, *J. Hyg. (Lond.)*, **64**, 105.

HOBBS, B. C. (1968) *Food Poisoning and Food Hygiene*, 2nd ed., London.

KINGSTON, D., LIDWELL, O. M., and WILLIAMS, R. E. O. (1962) The epidemiology of the common cold. II. The effect of ventilation, air disinfection and room size, *J. Hyg. (Lond.)*, **60**, 341.

LANCET (1970) Strategy of malaria eradication: a turning point?, Editorial, *Lancet*, **i**, 598.

MACLEOD, C. M. (1963) Biological implications of eradication and control, *Amer. Rev. resp. Dis.*, **88**, 763.

McENTEGART, M. G. (1969) Immunological tracing: bacteria, protozoa, helminths, fungi, in *Fluorescent Protein Tracing*, 3rd ed., ed. Nairn, R. C., Edinburgh (Chapter 7).

MILLER, D. L. (1970) The prophylactic and therapeutic uses of immunoglobulin in virus infections, in *Modern Trends in Medical Virology*, 2nd ed., eds. Heath, R. B., and Waterson, A. P., London.

MILLER, D. L., and GALBRAITH, N. S. (1965) Surveillance of the safety of oral poliomyelitis vaccine in England and Wales, 1962–4, *Brit. med. J.*, **2**, 504.

NATHANSON, N., and LANGMUIR, A. D. (1963) The Cutter incident. Poliomyelitis following formaldehyde—inactivated poliovirus vaccination in the United States during the spring of 1955, *Amer. J. Hyg.*, **78**, 16.

RAŠKA, K. (1966) National and international surveillance of communicable disease, *Chron. Wld Hlth Org.*, **20**, 428.

REPORT (1965) *Salmonellae in Cattle and their Feeding Stuffs, and the Relation to Human Infection*, a report of the Joint Working Party of the Veterinary Laboratory Services of the Ministry of Agriculture, Fisheries and Food, and the Public Health Laboratory Service, *J. Hyg. (Lond.)*, **63**, 223.

RIDLEY, M. (1959) Perineal carriage of *Staph. aureus*, *Brit. med. J.*, **1**, 270.

SCOTTISH HOME AND HEALTH DEPARTMENT (1964) *The Aberdeen Typhoid Outbreak, 1964*, Report of the Departmental Committee of Enquiry, Edinburgh Cmnd. 2542, H.M.S.O.

TAYLOR, C. E. D. (1969) Serological techniques, in *Automation and Data Processing in Pathology*, ed. Whitehead, T. P., *J. clin. Path.*, **22**, suppl. **3**, 14.

TUMOVA, B., SVANDOVA, E., and STUMPA, G. (1968) Findings of antibodies to animal influenza viruses in human sera and their significance for the study of interviral antigenic relationship, *J. Hyg. Epidem. (Praha)*, **12**, 284.

UNITED STATES NATIONAL CENTER FOR HEALTH STATISTICS (1963) *Origin, Program, and Operation of the U.S. National Health Survey*, Public Health Service Publication No. 1000, Series 1, No. 1, United States Department of Health, Education and Welfare, Washington D.C.

UNITED STATES PUBLIC HEALTH SERVICE (1969a) Surveillance summary. Measles—United States, 1968, *Morbid. and Mortal.*, **18**, 19.

UNITED STATES PUBLIC HEALTH SERVICE (1969b) Prelicensing statement on rubella virus vaccine. Recommendation of the Public Health Service Advisory Committee on Immunisation Practices, *Morbid. and Mortal.*, **18**, 124.

VERNON, E. (1969) Food poisoning and salmonella infections in England and Wales, 1967, *Publ. Hlth (Lond.)*, **83**, 205.

WILLIAMS, R. E. O., and TROTMAN, R. E. (1969) Automation in diagnostic bacteriology, in *Automation and Data Processing in Pathology*, ed. Whitehead, T. P., *J. clin. Path.*, **22**, suppl. **3**, 8.

WILSON, SIR GRAHAM S. (1962) Measles as a universal disease, *Amer. J. Dis. Child.*, **103**, 219.

WILSON, SIR GRAHAM S. (1967) *The Hazards of Immunisation*, London.

WORLD HEALTH ORGANIZATION (1968a) Fourteenth Report of the Expert Committee on Malaria, *Wld Hlth Org. techn Rep. Ser.*, No. 382.

WORLD HEALTH ORGANIZATION (1968b) *Smallpox Eradication*, Report of WHO Scientific Group, *Wld Hlth Org. techn. Rep. Ser.*, No. 393.

WORLD HEALTH ORGANIZATION (1968c) The surveillance of communicable diseases, *Chron. Wld Hlth Org.*, **22**, 439.

2

NON-COMMUNICABLE DISEASE

Neil Kessel

THE germ theory of disease has so permeated medical thinking that the term 'communicable disease' has been applied only to those conditions which arise by the transfer of a living agent from man to man or animal to man, sometimes through an intermediate host; but there are, of course, other modes of spread of illness in which there may well be communication of something not living from one host to another. Ideas can be communicated and give rise to illnesses: alcoholism, for example, and hysterical states may arise in this way; so may episodes of self-poisoning, even suicide. It is similarly the case with accidents, though it is, of course, the impulse to reckless driving which is communicated from youth to youth.

However, in the majority of instances of non-communicable disease with which the epidemiologist has been concerned there has genuinely been no communication. The spread of disease in a population is not from one case to another or from one living host to another, but to several people, due to an inanimate circumstance or occurrence in the environment. So, for instance, shortage of certain types of food causes avitaminoses, and air pollution gives rise to bronchitis.

In the past, few questions were asked about the epidemiology of such conditions, although there were some notable exceptions, for example in the field of nutritional disorders, and of goitre and cretinism. Rapid advances in the field of non-communicable disease have come about in the last twenty-five years, so that now a large proportion of epidemiological effort, particularly in the western world, is devoted to the study of non-infectious disease.

Some workers have used epidemiological techniques for 'completing the clinical picture', as Morris (1964) phrased it. They have sought for pre-symptomatic instances of the condition under study—examining whole populations for such states as *symptomless* hypertension (by sphygmomanometry) or *symptomless* diabetes mellitus (by urine and blood tests). Examination of uterine cervical smears for precancerous cells is an extension backwards from presymptomatic evidence of established disease to predisease evidence of disease. The term 'preclinical' is loosely used to denote either of these two significantly different things.

Can we assume that for every chronic disease there is a preclinical, and possibly a predisease state? If so, and if we then test a whole population (or a sample of it), we should find unrecognized individuals either with the disease or who will most probably develop it. The converse occurs where we have a specific test of immunity to the disease; those not immune will be at special risk. The secondary questions which follow are: 'Having discovered people with evidence of the disease who are going to develop it or who are at serious risk of developing it, can we do anything to resolve the situation?', and, 'What effect will any such action have on morbidity and mortality rates of the disease?' As McKeown (1968) puts it, in writing of screening procedures: 'There is a presumptive understanding, not merely that abnormality will be identified if it is present, but that those affected will derive benefit from subsequent treatment and care.' The epidemiologist's contribution would be to show a fall in morbidity or mortality rates because the condition had been presymptomatically detected. The value of various specific screening programmes is fully discussed in a Nuffield Provincial Hospitals Trust publication (1968).

Epidemiological investigation can sometimes help in the identification of disease syndromes. When two or more symptoms are often seen together this may be fortuitous, because both are common, or they may be aspects of the same disease. Suspected associations between, for example, chronic bronchitis and hypertension, or peptic ulcer and carcinoma of the stomach, might be investigated from this point of view. The two separate conditions do not have to be present in the individual person at the same time.

An extension of this idea has led to the development of the cluster theory of illness (Hinkle and Wolff, 1958; Hinkle et al., 1958). These workers found that, irrespective of the nature of the illnesses suffered, the temporal pattern of illnesses in an individual was not random; on the contrary, he was liable to a number of separate and apparently unrelated illnesses within a brief space of time. They related these periods to those of stress in life. This idea was followed up in a series of studies by Rahé, McKean, and Ransom (1967). Here, the temporal clustering was of clinically separate conditions. The same phenomenon, however, in relation to a single condition has led to the postulation of a possibly infective factor in diseases which were previously considered to be non-infective. This is especially so if the clustering can be demonstrated to occur in both space and time. Recently, such clustering has been shown for Burkitt's lymphoma (Pike, 1968).

To many epidemiologists aetiological questions are paramount, and this line of attack on non-communicable disease has certainly been fruitful. Broadly speaking, we ask whether some environmental feature is associated more often with the disease than would be expected by chance. The chance expectation is determined by reference to the frequency of the feature *either* in the whole population or in a random sample of it, *or else* by the examination of selected members of the population, a matched control group, chosen because they are like known sufferers in respect of other factors, such as age and sex, that are known to be relevant aetiologically.

Time relationships play an important part in such studies. We are all of us readily persuaded (rightly or wrongly) of a causal relationship between an environmental event and a clinical one if the former precedes the latter by a very short time. In non-communicable disease such a short time-span is relatively rare, except in violent deaths, but the London smog 'epidemic' of 1952 provides a good example (Ministry of Health, 1954). In most instances the time relationship is longer and the cause and effect significance correspondingly more difficult to demonstrate convincingly. In attempting to do this we may choose to begin our investigation either with the environmental occurrence or with the disease consequence, with the presumed cause or the presumed effect, with the earlier or the later event. Accordingly we work either forwards or backwards in time, making either a *prospective* or a *retrospective* inquiry [see CHAPTER 4].

Retrospective and prospective studies complement one another. The retrospective study usually precedes the prospective, perhaps because the question, 'What is the reason for this disease?' is more often asked in medicine than, 'What is the effect on disease rates of this environmental factor?' Retrospective studies are in general more easily mounted because there is a certainty of having a sufficient number of cases (measured by the 'effect' factor) and because they take less time and are usually less laborious. Thus, Doll and Hill (1950, 1952) carried out retrospective studies on patients suffering from carcinoma of the lung before they undertook their long-term prospective inquiry.

It is quite admissible for the 'effect' to have occurred before the subjects are first identified, but this effect should not be known to the research worker at the time he identifies the population for the prospective study. Here is an example: to see whether there was a high rate of suicide among alcoholics, a group of male patients treated for alcoholism some years previously was followed up to discover how many of them had subsequently killed themselves. Suicide is comparatively common, and the control group for this study consisted of the entire male population of Greater London, for whom the suicide rate is published. Age standardization was used, and both the cause and the effect, both the alcoholism and the suicide, had, in fact, already been recorded when the study was begun. But at the time the patients were selected for study the research worker did not know whether they were dead or not, and thus no bias was introduced into the results. The rate of suicide among alcoholics was found to be about 80 times the expected rate (Kessel and Grossman, 1961).

This type of study, which has been referred to as a 'prospective study in the past' or an 'historical prospective study', has been profitably used on a number of occasions. It has the considerable advantage that the waiting period between the environmental event and the development of the disease, which may be lengthy, has already occurred; the experimental study itself need not, therefore, take so long.

Where the group of subjects forming the experimental population in a prospective study is defined by their year of birth it is sometimes known as a 'cohort'. A cohort in popular English suggests an army moving forward; in Latin its definition is 'a multitude enclosed'; both meanings convey its epidemiological function. The cohort is marshalled and its progress is followed up. Douglas, for example, took a large representative sample of all children born in Great Britain during the first week of March, 1946. Later he studied their performance at school and various aspects of their health, in relation to their own characteristics at birth and to certain of their parents' characteristics (Douglas, 1960; Douglas, Ross, and Simpson, 1968).

Although a cohort is strictly defined by year of birth, the term is sometimes used to describe a group of individuals selected because they possess an abnormal characteristic in common. O'Neal and Robins (1958), for example, followed up a group of children attending a child guidance clinic between 1924 and 1929. The purposes of the two types of study differ slightly and the use of the term 'cohort' is probably better restricted to the former use— that of a group defined by birth date. This type of cohort analysis has been developed by Springett (1950), who referred to it as the generation method, and more recently by Case and Pearson (1957), and Harley and Hytten (1966).

Verification of a prediction, which occurs in a prospective inquiry, is undoubtedly more compelling than the discovery of an association from a retrospective study. Logically, however, the strength of the association may be no greater in the one case than in the other, and there is clearly a place for both types of inquiry. The development of mass data handling techniques should make us consider closely which would prove most fruitful for the particular investigation we might wish to undertake.

These techniques make possible the examination of the interrelationships between many more variables than was previously possible. In retrospective inquiries, for example, the use of the computer and multivariate analysis [see CHAPTERS 10 and 12 respectively] enables us to measure the relative strength of the associations between each of a large number of variables and the condition being studied. Similarly, in prospective studies, the significance can be found of the effects of many causal variables, singly or in combination, upon a large number of possible outcomes, where there are symptoms and illnesses. We are thus able to test many hypotheses simultaneously. This maximizes the number of questions we may ask in studies concerned either with cause factors of diseases or effect factors of environmental situations. An experiment involving a large number of subjects, and hence considerable labour, may have at its core the testing of a single hypothesis; nevertheless the 'pay-off' from the study may be considerably increased by collecting data from subjects concerning other possible aetiological factors, even though they may be irrelevant to the main hypothesis. Mass data handling techniques have enlarged our capacity to answer epidemiological questions to such an extent that we now need to examine our traditional, rather sparing, ways of asking these questions.

REFERENCES

CASE, R. A. M., and PEARSON, J. T. (1957) *Tables for Comparative Composite Cohort Analysis*, Studies on Medical and Population Subjects, No. 13, London, H.M.S.O.

DOLL, R., and HILL, A. B. (1950) Smoking and carcinoma of the lung. Preliminary report, *Brit. med. J.*, **2**, 739.

DOLL, R., and HILL, A. B. (1952) A study of the aetiology of carcinoma of the lung, *Brit. med. J.*, **2**, 1271.

DOUGLAS, J. W. B. (1960) 'Premature' children at primary schools, *Brit. med. J.*, **1**, 1008.

DOUGLAS, J. W. B., ROSS, J. M., and SIMPSON, H. R. (1968) *All Our Future*, London.

HARLEY, J. L., and HYTTEN, A. (1966) *Death rates by Site and Sex 1911–1920, Scotland*, Chester Beatty Institute, London.

HINKLE, L. E., JNR., and WOLFF, H. G. (1958) Ecologic investigations of the relationship between illness, life experiences and the social environment, *Ann. intern. Med.*, **49**, 1373.

HINKLE, L. E., JNR., CHRISTENSON, W. N., KAND, F. D., OSTFELD, A., THETFORD, W. N., and WOLFF, H. G. (1958) An investigation of the relation between life experience, personality characteristics and general susceptibility to illness, *Psychosom. Med.*, **20**, 278.

KESSEL, N., and GROSSMAN, G. (1961) Suicide in alcoholics, *Brit. med. J.*, **2**, 1671.

McKEOWN, T. (1968) Validation of screening procedures, in *Screening in Medical Care*, Nuffield Provincial Hospitals Trust, London, p. 2.

MINISTRY OF HEALTH (1954) *Mortality and Morbidity during the London Fog of December 1952*, Reports on Public Health and Medical Subjects, No. 95, London, H.M.S.O.

MORRIS, J. N. (1964) Completing the clinical picture, in *Uses of Epidemiology*, 2nd ed., Edinburgh, p. 110.

NUFFIELD PROVINCIAL HOSPITALS TRUST (1968) *Screening in Medical Care*, London.

O'NEAL, P., and ROBINS, LEE N. (1958) The relation of childhood behaviour problems to adult psychiatric studies, *Amer. J. Psychiat.*, **114**, 961.

PIKE, M. C. (1968) Detection of epidemicity with application to Burkitt's lymphoma and acute leukaemia, *Brit. J. prev. soc. Med.*, **22**, 114.

RAHÉ, R. H., McKEAN, J. D., JNR., and RANSOM, J. A. (1967) A longitudinal study of life-change and illness patterns, *J. psychosom. Res.*, **10**, 355.

SPRINGETT, V. H. (1950) Correspondence, *Lancet*, i, 926.

3

MEDICAL CARE

JOHN PEMBERTON

THE distribution of a disease in the population determines the nature and amount of preventive, diagnostic, and treatment services which are required and where they are required, so that anyone who is concerned with the provision of health services is obliged to inquire into this distribution. Epidemiologists have, therefore, become involved in the field of Medical Care or Health Services Administration, as it is sometimes called.

Medical care may be considered as the study and evaluation by epidemiological methods of the ways in which health services are, or could be, provided. Medical care studies can be applied to all types of health service whether preventive, diagnostic, therapeutic, or rehabilitative.

PREVENTIVE SERVICES

Communicable Disease: Preventive Trials

Before any prophylactic procedure is introduced for routine use, proper assessment of its safety and efficacy by means of controlled field trials is essential. Failure to do so can only result in protracted uncertainty about its value. For many years this was the fate of BCG (Hart, 1967) and it was not until sixty years after typhoid vaccine was introduced that the first adequate assessment of its protective effect was made, in the trials of the Yugoslav Typhoid Commission (1962). The need for adequate field trials of any new vaccine is now recognized as an indispensable prerequisite of its release for general use. Examples are the extensive trials that were made of poliomyelitis and measles vaccines (Medical Research Council, 1957, 1968).

The principles governing the conduct of such trials, in which the epidemiologist has a central role, have been set out in a monograph published by the World Health Organization (Pollock, 1966). This monograph begins by suggesting that the problems involved in determining the value of a vaccine for man can usually be condensed into a single question: 'How safe and effective will it be in the environment in which it is used?' The question of safety is undoubtedly paramount. No vaccine is acceptable unless the hazards of giving it are very substantially less than those of the natural disease. The first aim of a field trial, therefore, is to identify the risks to vaccinees, to define contraindications to vaccination, and to determine which groups of patients may be specially susceptible to adverse reactions. When using live vaccines, the chances of spread to contacts of vaccinees with the risk of causing disease, due to reactivation of virulence, also have to be assessed. The second question, that of efficacy, is not simply a matter of whether the vaccine can protect against disease but whether it will do so to a useful degree in the persons whom it is desired to protect. The aim of a trial, therefore, should be to measure the degree of protection that can be expected under the circumstances in which the vaccine is intended to be used. Where there is an alternative in the type of vaccine and route of administration, for example between live attenuated and killed virus polio vaccines, the question of which vaccine is most appropriate may also arise.

Field trials designed to assess efficacy and safety must be carefully planned. It is essential for the trial to be conducted in vaccinated and control groups which are fully comparable; to ensure this they should be allocated at random from the same population. Without this precaution it is impossible to be certain that adverse reactions which might be attributable to the vaccine are not simply chance observations that could have occurred without vaccination. The measurement of protective efficacy depends on a comparison between illness attack rates in vaccinated and unvaccinated persons. This is only valid if the two groups are exposed to the same risks of infection with the agent concerned and have the same capacity to resist disease. Numbers included in the trial must be sufficient to obtain a statistically significant difference in attack rates between the two groups, given the expected attack rate in unimmunized persons and the minimum of protection required. Wherever possible, trials should be supported by laboratory investigations, which will determine whether or not the subjects have been infected and the antibody response to vaccination.

There are also a number of subsidiary questions to be answered by field trials which affect the planning of immunization schedules. The number and spacing of doses of vaccine to obtain the optimum antibody response and the duration of immunity need to be determined. The age at which vaccination is carried out may influence the response: some vaccines are ineffective if given in early infancy, as maternal antibody may interfere in the response. Giving more than one vaccine simultaneously may reduce the antibody response and increase the risk of reactions; thus, when a new vaccine is introduced this is a matter that requires investigation before recommendations on schedules can be made.

Questions concerning the efficacy and safety of vaccines do not end with satisfactory field trials. It is essential that there should be provision for continuing surveillance. The protective efficacy of a vaccine may alter, due to changes in the prevalent antigenic variant of the organism concerned, and reactions, if very rare or delayed, may only be detectable after a prolonged interval. Moreover, with changing disease incidence, the need for vaccination may alter, and the benefits to the health of the community must be critically reassessed from time to time. For all these reasons, surveillance must be a permanent feature of any vaccination programme.

Non-communicable Disease Prevention

In the field of non-communicable disease the possibilities of prevention are at present fewer than those for communicable disease; investigations of their effectiveness are therefore less common.

The prevention of nutritional diseases by specific social measures provides examples of a preventive service in the field of non-communicable disease, the effectiveness of which is capable of assessment by epidemiological inquiry. Clearly it is in a nation's economic interest if the minimum effective amount of a dietary supplement required to prevent a nutritional disease can be determined, whether this supplement is iodide in table salt to prevent goitre or dried milk to prevent kwashiorkor. Studies to determine the effectiveness of national food policies in relation to the prevalence of nutritional disease, particularly in countries where these are still common, are clearly of great value. For example, experiments carried out by a Medical Research Council team during the Second World War to determine the minimum human requirements of Vitamins A and C were of this type (Medical Research Council, 1949 and 1953). More recently Elwood et al. (1968) and Elwood (1968) have reported a series of experiments to try and determine the effectiveness of the iron which is by law added to flour in the United Kingdom as a method of preventing iron deficiency anaemia in the community.

Today, however, in the more affluent countries, problems of nutritional deficiency have become much less important, while the problem of obesity is causing increasing concern. Unlike dietary deficiency in populations, obesity is a condition for which the State can do little, and the remedy and prevention would seem to lie in the hands of the individual. Indeed, it is becoming increasingly clear that the prevention of several of the more important causes of illness and death, particularly in the western world today, lie in the realm of human behaviour. It follows that the medical care epidemiologist working in the field of preventive services will in the future be concerned with the success or otherwise of steps taken to bring about such changes in human behaviour.

The series of papers by Doll and Hill (1964) on the relationship of cigarette smoking to lung cancer in doctors illustrates how a certain type of behaviour can increase the risk of developing a disease and, conversely, how the abandonment of a habit may bring about a decrease in mortality (Doll, 1966). In this case the change in behaviour was, presumably, brought about because a knowledge of the dangers of cigarette smoking persuaded many doctors to give up the habit. It would be valuable to discover why many doctors have changed their behaviour in this respect—and, moreover, why some have not done so. The explanation for the different reaction among doctors to facts which must be known to all of them is presumably to be found in differences of motivation and personality. Thus, the epidemiologist investigating problems in medical care is increasingly concerned with the behavioural sciences, and can obtain valuable help from the psychologist and social scientist in investigating questions of this sort.

Changes in behaviour related to health or safety are sometimes brought about by a change in the law such as the introduction of compulsory vaccination against smallpox or the introduction of the 30 m.p.h. speed limit in towns. A recent example of a remarkable change in behaviour resulting from legislation in Great Britain was the change in motoring habits which followed the introduction of the law making it an offence to drive with a concentration of alcohol in the blood greater than 80 mg per 100 ml. In the year following the introduction of this legislation the number of deaths on the road declined by about 1,200 or approximately 20 per cent from the previous year.

It would be useful to know what particular changes in behaviour took place which were relevant to this result. What sort of people changed their behaviour and what sort did not? Are the changes in behaviour being maintained, and if not, why not? Questions relating to the effectiveness of legislation such as this, designed to prevent disease or accidents, are very appropriate for epidemiological inquiry.

One of the prerequisites of such inquiries is an abundant supply of ongoing routinely collected data concerning illnesses, accidents, and deaths in defined populations and, in addition, data about changes in behaviour. Indirect methods of estimating such changes can be employed, such as the examination of trends in tobacco or alcohol consumption, in the number of licensed vehicles on the roads, in the illegitimacy rate, in the prevalence of venereal disease, crime and delinquency, drug addiction, mental illness and mental subnormality, and suicide. As long ago as 1933 Lidbetter showed that there existed a subgroup in the population which he referred to as the 'social problem group' in which 'anti-social' behavioural patterns tended to overlap. What is now needed for epidemiological studies of behaviour in relation to disease is a much greater degree of linkage of records, so that the relationships between patterns of behaviour, and disease and accidents can be investigated.

The future prevention of diseases and accidents resulting wholly or in part from habits and ways of living is likely to depend largely upon successful health education. An important task of the epidemiologist interested in this field, therefore, is to measure the effectiveness of different types of health education. The following type of question is relevant: 'With a given expenditure of money and manpower, would a greater effect be obtained in reducing the amount of cigarette smoking by 15-year-old schoolchildren, by showing them an anti-smoking film or by giving them a talk illustrated by slides?' Cvjetanovic (1958) carried out studies of this sort in Yugoslavia comparing the effectiveness of sound films, silent films, and talks in persuading village people to accept typhoid inoculation.

Cartwright, Martin, and Thomson (1960) in a study of the efficacy of an anti-smoking campaign in Edinburgh concluded that 'Campaigns of this type are unlikely to produce changes in behaviour except possibly in an indirect and long-term fashion'. Holland and Elliott (1968) also reported disappointing results. Clearly, however, this type of investigation is very necessary if the effectiveness of health education is to be increased.

Possibly one of the reasons for the slow development of health education and the relatively small amount of support it has received from some governments and from the medical profession in general is that so few studies have been made demonstrating its effectiveness.

The routine administration of drugs on a mass scale, such as serum cholesterol reducing drugs for the prevention of coronary artery disease, is now a possibility in the future, and the measurement of the effectiveness and risks associated with such preventive measures is a task for the epidemiologist. Such studies have already been carried out in relation to the use of oral contraceptives, and some have demonstrated their risks (Vessey and Doll, 1969). An efficient monitoring system in which records of administration of drugs used for prevention are linked with records of the occurrence of the condition they are supposed to prevent, and with the occurrence of side effects, will be needed to answer questions relating to the effectiveness and safety of such procedures.

There are few services organized as yet for the prevention of congenital disease. The epidemiologist could perhaps contribute to the prevention of these conditions by helping in the development of early warning systems for detecting changes in the prevalence of congenital defects in order to identify at the earliest possible moment the 'thalidomide' type of epidemic.

DIAGNOSTIC PROCEDURES

Epidemiologists, when carrying out field prevalence surveys, have, in order to be able to count cases, sometimes been forced, because of the unavailability of specific laboratory or X-ray tests, to define the disease under study by a selection of its chief symptoms. This requirement led to the discovery that experienced observers may vary to a larger extent than expected in their interpretation of the same clinical phenomena, and, further, that a single investigator may give a different interpretation of the same phenomenon after a period of time (Oldham, 1968).

Questions relating to observer variation or error are therefore of concern to the epidemiologist, and their existence and magnitude should be investigated at the outset of any epidemiological inquiry. Because of difficulties associated with observer variation, epidemiologists have encouraged the development and use of portable apparatus for field surveys capable of making objective measurements, for example a sphygmomanometer (Rose, Holland, and Crowley, 1964), and a spirometer (McDermott, McDermott, and Collins, 1968). Such instruments have proved of great value in epidemiological studies, but before they are introduced into an investigation the following questions should be asked:

1. Is the information the instrument provides relevant to the question being asked?
2. Is the measurement reproducible?
3. Does the measurement discriminate between normals and abnormals reasonably well?

In developing objective diagnostic tests for use in clinical surveys and in the formulation of definitions of disease for the purpose of such surveys, epidemiologists have made an important contribution to greater precision in clinical diagnosis.

Epidemiological population surveys have also led to considerable questioning of accepted 'normal' values for many quantitative diagnostic tests, for example the normal range of haemoglobin concentrations. Much work remains to be done in the field of establishing normal ranges in the population in different age–sex groups, in giving 'probability of being abnormal' values with regard to levels outside 'the normal range', and in establishing the levels at which treatment should be given.

The development of diagnostic screening procedures raises a number of important epidemiological questions. Some are of considerable epidemiological interest: for example, 'What are the prevalence rates of the condition being screened for in the community and in subgroups of the community?' There are also technical questions to be answered such as: 'What is the proportion of false positives and false negatives?'; and, most important of all, 'What is the effect of the screening programme on the morbidity and mortality rates of the population from the disease in question?' An important question to answer before embarking on a screening programme is whether anything useful can be done about any abnormalities which are likely to be discovered. Many observations are needed to evaluate screening programmes in terms of subsequent morbidity and mortality; the linkage of screening data with morbidity and mortality data on a national scale would greatly facilitate the evaluation of these procedures.

TREATMENT

It is questionable whether the assessment of the effectiveness of a new type of medical or surgical treatment lies in the province of the epidemiologist. In our opinion the controlled clinical trial is a problem for the clinician and medical statistician rather than the epidemiologist. On the other hand the epidemiologist should be concerned with estimating needs for treatment services based on epidemiological data and with giving advice about the best way of providing such a service.

An example of the sort of question which can be investigated with advantage is: 'How many beds for a certain speciality, for example geriatrics, are required for a city with a population of half a million?'

Clearly numerous subsidiary questions need to be answered first, such as:

1. What is the age distribution of the population, and in what way and how fast is this changing?

2. What is the need for geriatric hospital beds at different ages over 60? (This would require a population survey.)

3. For what illnesses must provision be made? What sort of provision?

4. What is their prognosis and duration?

5. What are the attitudes of the old people and their relatives to hospital care?

6. Can the beds be staffed even if provided?

Hospital beds are expensive to establish and maintain, and some valuable medical care epidemiology has been done in the study of bed usage. Various studies have shown that there are wide differences between countries in duration of hospital stay for the same conditions, and between hospitals too (Heasman, 1964; Pearson *et al.*, 1968). Other studies have shown that patients may recover as well after a short stay as after a longer stay in hospital, for example, after hernia operations (Morris, Ward, and Handyside, 1968).

The team which worked on the problem of tuberculosis in Madras (Lancet, 1961) showed that domiciliary treatment could be as effective as hospital treatment, that it was possible to treat many more cases in this way, and that the cost per case was then much lower.

Where comprehensive national health services exist and drugs are prescribed on a statutory form, the possibility arises of answering a number of important questions about drug usage. If information about the type and quantity of drug prescribed is stored in a form suitable for computer analysis, drug usage by geographical areas can be studied using large quantities of data. Wade (1968) has published data relating to the prescription of certain drugs in different parts of Northern Ireland and at different times, which was derived

D

from computer storage and analysis of all National Health Service prescriptions in Northern Ireland.

Questions about the need for rehabilitation, for services for the handicapped, and for the care of the dying can all be approached from the epidemiological point of view.

USE OF EXISTING RECORDS OR AN AD HOC SURVEY

Sometimes, records are already available for abstract and analysis in medical care problems—for example, records of schoolchildren with physical or mental handicaps. Often, however, an *ad hoc* field survey must be undertaken.

Many surveys have been conducted in the past because it has been suspected that the medical needs of a particular population group, such as those over 65 years of age, were not being fully met. The results are often presented in tables showing the prevalence of defects and of needs expressed as percentages in subgroups of age, sex, civil state, and social class.

If the sample is truly random, the tables enable estimates of prevalences and needs to be made for the whole community. Often in the past they have revealed an unexpectedly high prevalence of disabilities and unmet needs for treatment. Sheldon's survey of old people in Wolverhampton (1948) provides an early example of this sort of study; the information obtained from them is of considerable value to those responsible for planning and administering central and local health services.

There are clearly an unlimited number of questions relating to medical care which require an epidemiological approach in order to be solved. Some of these can, and should, be investigated by the authorities responsible for providing the services, particularly, perhaps, those questions which lie within the areas of effectiveness in relation to cost, and of organization and methods. Competent epidemiologists interested in the field of medical care are rare, and they should not therefore be called upon to investigate questions which a good administrator, perhaps with some epidemiological advice and statistical help, can tackle.

The future success of epidemiological research in relation to medical care problems is likely to be closely related to the quality, content, and availability of medical records. The value of a medical record is sometimes assessed according to the amount of detail it contains, and from the clinical point of view this is undoubtedly important. Some clinical records, however, become so voluminous that they defeat their own end because no one has time to find the particular fact that is wanted in the mass of information provided. For the epidemiologist, records must be easily accessible in large numbers and there must be no doubt about the identification of the individual. Moreover, the recording of negative findings is as important as that of positive ones. The basic data he usually requires include the date of birth, sex, occupation, address, diagnosis, duration of illness, time off work or stay in hospital, and whether the illness was fatal or not.

Thus, we see that a great many questions in the fields of medical care and epidemiology could be answered if this basic information for all medically treated illness in a community were recorded, coded, and stored in a form suitable for computer analysis.

REFERENCES

CARTWRIGHT, A., MARTIN, F. M., and THOMPSON, J. G. (1960) Efficacy of an anti-smoking campaign, *Lancet*, **i**, 327.

CVJETANOVIC, B. (1958) The evaluation of some different methods of health education in Yugoslavia (Appendix 3), in *Recent Studies in Epidemiology*, eds. Pemberton, J., and Willard, H., Oxford, p. 198.

DOLL, R., and HILL, A. B. (1964) Mortality in relation to smoking: ten years of observations of British doctors, *Brit. med. J.*, **1**, 1399.

DOLL, R. (1966) Lung cancer and tobacco, *Bronches*, **16**, 313.

ELWOOD, P. C., NEWTON, D., EAKINS, J. D., and BROWN, D. A. (1968) Absorption of iron from bread, *Amer. J. clin. Nutr.*, **21**, 1162.

ELWOOD, P. C. (1968) *Studies of the Absorption of Iron from Bread*, report of the panel on iron in flour, London, H.M.S.O.

HART, P. D'A. (1967) Efficacy and applicability of mass BCG vaccination in tuberculosis control, *Brit. med. J.*, **1**, 587.

HEASMAN, M. A. (1964) How long in hospital?, *Lancet*, **ii**, 539.

HOLLAND, W. W., and ELLIOTT, A. (1968) Cigarette smoking, respiratory symptoms and anti-smoking propaganda, *Lancet*, **i**, 41.

LANCET (LEADING ARTICLE) (1961) The Madras experiment, *Lancet*, **ii**, 532.

LIDBETTER, E. J. (1933) *Heredity and the Social Problem Group*, London.

MEDICAL RESEARCH COUNCIL (1949) *Vitamin A Requirements of Human Adults*, Special Report Series No. 264, London, H.M.S.O.

MEDICAL RESEARCH COUNCIL (1953) *Vitamin C Requirements of Human Adults*, Special Report Series No. 280, London, H.M.S.O.

MEDICAL RESEARCH COUNCIL (1957) The assessment of the British vaccine against poliomyelitis. A report to the Medical Research Council by its Poliomyelitis Vaccines Committee, *Brit. med. J.*, **1**, 1271.

MEDICAL RESEARCH COUNCIL (1968) Vaccination against measles: clinical trial of live measles vaccine given alone and live vaccine preceded by killed vaccine. Second report to the Medical Research Council by the Measles Vaccines Committee, *Brit. med. J.*, **2**, 449.

McDERMOTT, M., McDERMOTT, T. J., and COLLINS, M. M. (1968) A portable bellows spirometer and timing unit for the measurement of respiratory function, *Med. biol. Engng*, **6**, 291.

MORRIS, D., WARD, A. W. M., and HANDYSIDE, A. J. (1968) Early discharge after hernia repair, *Lancet*, **i**, 681.

OLDHAM, P. D. (1968) Observer error in medicine, *Proc. roy. Soc. Med.*, **61**, 447.

PEARSON, R. J. C., SMEDBY, B., BERFENSTAM, R., LOGAN, R. F. L., BURGESS, A. M., and PETERSEN, O. (1968) Hospital caseloads in Liverpool, New England and Uppsala—an international comparison, *Lancet*, **ii**, 559.

POLLOCK, T. M. (1966) Trials of prophylactic agents for the control of communicable disease. A guide to their organisation and evaluation, *Wld Hlth Org. Monogr. Ser.*, No. 52.

ROSE, G. A., HOLLAND, W. W., and CROWLEY, E. A. (1964) A sphygmomanometer for epidemiologists, *Lancet*, **i**, 296.

SHELDON, J. H. (1948) *The Social Medicine of Old Age*, Nuffield Foundation, London.

VESSEY, M. P., and DOLL, R. (1969) Investigation of relation between use of oral contraceptives and thrombo embolic disease, *Brit. med. J.*, **2**, 651.

WADE, O. L. (1968) The computer and drug prescribing, in *Computers in the Service of Medicine*, Nuffield Provincial Hospitals Trust, London.

YUGOSLAV TYPHOID COMMISSION (1962) A controlled field trial of the effectiveness of phenol and alcohol typhoid vaccines, *Bull. Wld Hlth Org.*, **26**, 357.

PART II

STUDY DESIGN

4

PRINCIPLES OF STUDY DESIGN

W. W. HOLLAND

AN epidemiological inquiry studies a condition in relation to its aetiology, natural history, and distribution in the population. Although all three topics are fundamental to an understanding of a condition, a single investigation will clearly be unable to reveal detailed information on each one of them. The epidemiologist is therefore faced at the very outset of his inquiry with the problem of defining the specific purpose of his study.

Once the aim of the study has been established, the second task of the investigator is to choose his study population. A group of female office workers, for example, would be unlikely to be involved in a study of the causes of pneumoconiosis; this would clearly be undertaken among an occupational group exposed to dust hazard. The absurdity of this situation illustrates a fundamental principle of epidemiology: the need to define the area of study and to relate this to the aim of the investigation.

The aim of a study also governs its form and method—that is, its design. Various techniques have now been evolved for the epidemiological study of a particular condition, and this chapter is intended to outline the different approaches currently in use. All the techniques described here are illustrated by reference to the study of one condition, chronic bronchitis. There are several reasons for the choice of this condition: it is common in most countries of the world, its prevalence is well documented, and a number of investigations have been undertaken into the aetiology of the disease. Previous studies of chronic bronchitis therefore serve to demonstrate both the different techniques used in epidemiology and the principal sources of data available to the epidemiologist. The latter will be discussed in greater detail in later chapters.

MORTALITY AND MORBIDITY STATISTICS

In CHAPTER 5 the possible sources of routinely collected mortality and morbidity figures are outlined. The methods of collection are described, and the problems which arise from a consideration of these data are indicated. Although the remarks have a general application to all conditions, they are clearly also relevant to the specific study of chronic bronchitis.

An examination of mortality and morbidity statistics demonstrates the frequency of a condition in different age, sex, social class, and nationality groups. For chronic bronchitis, mortality figures from different countries of the world show that the disease is more common in Britain than elsewhere. Moreover, the mortality figures for Britain show that chronic bronchitis is more often found in older than in younger age groups, is more common in males than in females, and occurs more frequently in lower social class groups and in urban areas. Morbidity statistics for England and Wales reflect a similar pattern (Holland, 1965).

The conclusions one can draw from these trends are, however, few, since most chronic conditions occur in older people, and the many factors which contribute to the differences between towns and rural areas render any broad distinction between the two types of environment unhelpful. No ready explanation is available for the sex and social class differences. It is therefore impossible to obtain any clear understanding of the aetiology of the condition from these sources, and it is consequently equally impossible to justify the choice of any course of preventive action from findings derived from them.

The major deficiency of studies of mortality and morbidity statistics is that they can give no idea of the personal characteristics of the individual which may influence the development of the disease. In order to obtain this knowledge, a personal examination of relatively few subjects is required. In a study of the development of chronic bronchitis there is also the additional problem of the long evolution of the disease. The onset of this condition can, in the majority of cases, be traced back to early life, and this inevitably complicates any study of its aetiology.

Studies of mortality and morbidity statistics do, however, demonstrate the frequency of the disease in different age–sex groups and in individuals living in different areas; hypotheses about the aetiology of the disease may be suggested on the basis of these figures. These hypotheses may be refined by the examination of a number of subjects, for example in a case-control study.

Case-control studies

A case-control study is possibly the simplest technique available for the study of individual subjects. In this type of study the number of patients with a disease are matched with an equal number of individuals without it who are broadly comparable (for example, in age and sex) to the first group. Data is collected from both groups on any personal or environmental characteristics which might be thought to contribute to the development of the disease. Questionnaires may, for example, provide information on place of birth, area of residence, occupation, social class, number of children, marital status, smoking habits, and alcohol consumption. The relative frequency with which each of these factors occurs in both groups is then determined. If certain factors predominate among the group with the condition, this indicates an association which may be causal.

Case-control studies have demonstrated quite clearly that individuals with chronic bronchitis tend to smoke more heavily than those without it. Such retrospective studies have, however, failed to determine the relative importance of this and other factors in the aetiology of the condition.

Longitudinal Studies

Once the importance of cigarette smoking in the development of chronic bronchitis has been established, the next step is to concentrate on a group of individuals of varying smoking habits, including non-smokers, and to follow this group over a period of years. The rate of occurrence, or incidence, of chronic bronchitis in the study group is assessed, and any patterns of morbidity or mortality which appear may be examined in relation to their smoking habits. This type of study is called a longitudinal or prospective study. Its principal value is that any one factor may be examined in detail and the magnitude of risks estimated. It will, for example, be possible to determine whether those who smoke have a greater tendency to develop the condition than those who do not, and whether those who smoke heavily are more liable to develop the condition than those who smoke less.

The investigations by Doll and Hill (1956) and Doll (1959) into the smoking habits of doctors provide classic examples of this prospective method of inquiry. These studies made an invaluable contribution to the understanding of the aetiology of lung cancer, since they clearly demonstrated an increased risk among cigarette smokers as opposed to cigar smokers, pipe smokers or non-smokers. The risk was also shown to be directly related to the number of cigarettes smoked.

Although this method is extremely valuable where some of the principal factors involved in the development of the disease have already been identified and a precise hypothesis about its aetiology has already been formulated, it has serious disadvantages where previous knowledge about the disease is less clearly defined. Only a proportion of the original group actually develop the disease, and it is necessary to study a large population for a short period of time or a smaller population for a longer period in order to draw valid conclusions from the results. It is therefore difficult to study the influence of more than one factor in any one study, though other factors, which may or may not be known to the investigator, could be involved in the development of the disease. It is, then, impossible to gain a comprehensive picture of the aetiology of a condition, or to establish the importance of new factors in a prospective study.

Some of the problems involved in prospective studies are discussed by Doll (1964), and the difficulties found in the planning of a prospective study are described by Waters and Elwood [CHAPTER 6]. With the increasing availability of computers and recent developments in methods of record linkage [CHAPTERS 7 and 8], it is, however, very probable that such studies will in the future become relatively easy to execute. By studying large groups one may then be able to standardize for the influence of one factor, in order to estimate the risk for other possible factors. This may also enable one to assess the relative magnitude of risk for each of the several factors involved.

Cross-sectional Studies

A cross-sectional or prevalence study aims to determine either the proportion of people affected by one or more conditions or the frequency distribution of different levels of one or more quantitative attributes (for example, weight or arterial pressure) within a defined population at a particular point in time (after Fletcher and Oldham, 1964).

A cross-sectional study, like the longitudinal type, tests a hypothesis suggested by mortality and/or case-control studies. These have demonstrated that chronic bronchitis is more common in particular age–sex groups and is related to area of residence and to cigarette smoking. Several hypotheses may now be formulated from these findings, but for the purposes of this chapter two contradictory theories will be considered. The first is that area of residence contributes to the aetiology of chronic bronchitis independently of personal factors such as cigarette smoking and occupation; the second is that area of residence is unimportant in the aetiology of the disease, but that occupation does contribute to its development. Different types of study design are required to test the two hypotheses.

An examination of the first hypothesis—that the influence of area of residence acts independently of other known factors—requires that the study population should be drawn from the same occupational group but from different areas. Two recent studies in Great Britain (Holland and Reid, 1965) and the United States (Holland et al., 1965) have followed this pattern. In an examination of individuals doing the same work but living in different areas, information on respiratory symptoms was obtained by questionnaire, measurements of lung function were made using simple portable techniques, and samples of sputum were collected. From this evidence the authors were able to demonstrate that, among individuals of the same occupation, differences found in the frequency of chronic bronchitic symptoms and levels of ventilatory function were related both to area of residence and to smoking habits. The influence of area of residence was also shown to be independent of smoking, since in certain areas the frequency and severity of respiratory disturbance was found to be consistently higher for groups of similar smoking habits.

An examination of the second hypothesis—that occupation is an overriding factor in the development of chronic bronchitis—requires the study of individuals of different occupations living in the same area. In one such study (Lowe, 1969), an examination of respiratory symptoms and lung function among steel workers in South Wales failed to demonstrate that occupation, independent of smoking habits, had a major effect on the development of the condition.

DEFINING THE ONSET OF THE CONDITION

The problem of chronic bronchitis is principally confined to the middle and older age groups, but as it was stated earlier, the aetiological investigation of the disease is complicated by its long evolution. In order to assess all possible factors which could contribute to the development of the condition it is necessary to determine when the disease starts. This problem may be approached in a variety of ways, using any one of the study techniques described above. Middle-aged individuals with chronic bronchitis may, for example, be questioned about their past medical history (a retrospective survey). This is, however, a poor method of defining the onset of the disease; evidence wholly dependent on recall is, in fact, suspect in all studies. An alternative method of inquiry is to study a group of subjects prospectively from childhood to middle-age. This, however, is an extremely time-consuming task, and the organization of data collection would present many difficulties using present methods. Record linkage systems such as those described by Heasman and Massé [CHAPTERS 7 and 8] may nevertheless make such studies possible in future.

At present, the only practicable method of determining the importance of childhood experience in the later development of chronic respiratory disease is to carry out a prevalence study of respiratory symptoms and conditions in children. In a study in Kent all children in certain age groups resident and attending school in four areas of the county were examined for evidence of respiratory symptoms and depression of lung function (Holland et al., 1969). Details of past respiratory illness were obtained from questionnaires completed by the parents. The results of this study demonstrate the independent effect of the following factors in the prevalence of respiratory symptoms and impaired ventilatory function: area of residence, smoking habits, social class, and past history of respiratory illness. It is, therefore, possible to assume that these influences begin to act early in life, and that effective preventive action should be taken in childhood and early adult life, rather than in middle-age when the need for medical treatment first becomes apparent.

MEDICAL CARE AND THE UTILIZATION OF MEDICAL
SERVICES

The studies discussed above have illustrated a number of possible approaches to the study of the aetiology of chronic bronchitis. Epidemiology is now becoming increasingly concerned with two further questions: 'What effect, if any, does medical care have on the evolution of a particular disease?'

and, 'What facilities are available for the care of individuals with this condition?' The study techniques used in aetiological investigations are equally applicable to an examination of these problems.

In a retrospective inquiry, for example, a study could be made of a group of hospital in-patients, in an attempt to determine where the patients come from and what care they are receiving. Since all the subjects are, however, receiving treatment, this type of inquiry fails to answer problems concerned with the need for medical services or the utilization of services in different groups of the population.

In order to answer these questions it is necessary to study a section of the total population. The simplest method of achieving this would be to identify a study population by census, to ask all members of the population what symptoms they have and to assess the care they have received. But this is an uneconomic method of inquiry, since it fails to take into account social class differences in both the utilization of medical care and the prevalence of a condition. Cartwright (1964) has suggested that individuals from different social class groups may use medical facilities in different ways, and chronic bronchitis has been shown to be more common in lower than in higher social class groups. Important age and sex differences have also been found.

In order to study sufficient numbers of cases from all sections of the population, it is therefore advisable to take a random sample of the population stratified according to age, sex, and social class. Since the disease is uncommon among young people one must draw a larger proportion of these individuals in the sample. A larger number of women than men, and a greater proportion of the higher than the lower social class groups should also be included in the study of the group. Bennett and Kasap [CHAPTER 9] describe how the selection of the appropriate sampling fractions may be achieved. If this method of selection is employed, it is possible to study groups large enough to make valid comparisons while limiting the size of the original sample group.

One further refinement is possible in the selection of a sample group for the study of the utilization of medical services. As we have seen, only a small number of individuals in the population have chronic bronchitis, and time and resources will be wasted if too many of those without the condition are included in the sample population. A two-stage inquiry process may therefore be adopted: at the first stage individuals with the condition are identified; in the second an assessment is made of the use which these individuals have made of the medical services available.

It may be argued that the investigator could by-pass the first stage of this process by studying only those individuals known to be suffering from chronic bronchitis. It is, however, clearly inadequate to study only hospital populations, since various selection factors (for example, the severity of the disease, area of residence, and the attitude of the patient's general practitioner) have been shown to operate on the cases treated in both in- and out-patient departments. (Bennett, 1966; Montgomery, 1968; Palmer *et al.*, 1969). An alternative approach would be to study a general practice group with chronic bronchitis. This would provide a more representative sample of the total population, but as Morrell (personal communication) has recently demonstrated, the age–sex register of a general practitioner is often inaccurate, as a proportion of individuals on the list are no longer resident in the area. This would be unimportant if the loss were equal in all age–sex groups, but the author has shown that the loss varies according to both age and sex. One must therefore accept that conclusions based on general practice registers are not entirely valid, and that there is no substitute for general population studies.

This chapter has described the different ways in which epidemiological studies of a particular condition may be designed. An attempt has been made to assess the relative merits of each type of inquiry, and to show the way in which the method of study chosen should be related to the aim of the study. It should be remembered that these techniques may be applied to the examination of any condition, whether acute or chronic.

REFERENCES

BENNETT, A. E. (1966) Case selection in a London teaching hospital, *Med. Care*, **4**, 138.

CARTWRIGHT, A. (1964) The influence of social class, in *Human Relations and Hospital Care*, London.

DOLL, R. (1959) Lung cancer and cigarette smoking, *Acta Un. int. Cancr.*, **15**, 417.

DOLL, R. (1964) Retrospective and prospective studies, in *Medical Surveys and Clinical Trials*, 2nd ed., ed. Witts, L. J., London, p. 71.

DOLL, R., and HILL, A. B. (1956) Lung cancer and other causes of death in relation to smoking, *Brit. med. J.*, **2**, 1011.

FLETCHER, C. M., and OLDHAM, P. D. (1964) Prevalence surveys, in *Medical Surveys and Clinical Trials*, 2nd ed., ed. Witts, L. J., London, p. 50.

HOLLAND, W. W. (1965) The rationale of field surveys, *Milbank mem. Fd Quart.*, **43**, Part 2, 77.

HOLLAND, W. W., and REID, D. D. (1965) The urban factor in chronic bronchitis, *Lancet*, i, 445.

HOLLAND, W. W., REID, D. D., SELTSER, R., and STONE, R. W. (1965) Respiratory disease in England and the United States. Studies of comparative prevalence, *Arch. environm. Hlth*, **10**, 338.

HOLLAND, W. W., HALIL, T., BENNETT, A. E., and ELLIOTT, A. (1969) Factors influencing the onset of chronic respiratory disease, *Brit. med. J.*, **3**, 205.

LOWE, C. R. (1969) Industrial bronchitis, *Brit. med. J.*, **1**, 465.

MONTGOMERY, K. M. (1968) Out-patients of a London teaching hospital, *Brit. J. prev. soc. Med.*, **22**, 50.

PALMER, J. W., KASAP, H. S., BENNETT, A. E., and HOLLAND, W. W. (1969) The use of hospitals by a defined population, *Brit. J. prev. soc. Med.*, **23**, 91.

PART III

COLLECTION OF DATA

5

COLLECTION OF DATA FROM ESTABLISHED SOURCES

K. Uemura

In almost all countries of the world there exists at least some system of routine collection of data in which epidemiologists are interested. Population censuses and civil registration systems provide valuable background data in many epidemiological studies. Morbidity statistics derived from systems for the notification of disease and from medical services are often the subject of epidemiological study by themselves, while in studies of a different kind these readily available data often direct epidemiologists' attention to the fields requiring further research.

However, there is a wide disparity among the countries of the world in the availability of basic statistical data. Civil registration systems, for instance, from which vital statistics are derived, have already been in operation for several centuries in Europe. On the other hand, there are still a number of countries in the world in which no such system exists. Although there is no doubt that the importance will be recognized of legally establishing the citizenship, entitlements, and obligations of each individual in those countries, it will take many more decades before a permanent civil registration system is established in all parts of the world.

A number of difficulties also arise in more developed countries in connection with routine data collection systems. Many of these systems are operated in conformity with firmly established legal provisions and traditions, involving considerable size of administrative organization and the handling of voluminous statistical data. In spite of rapidly changing health requirements, it is not easy to adapt the systems to cope with the needs of those who use statistics. Furthermore, because of the huge population to be covered and the large staff engaged, it is often difficult to achieve and maintain a satisfactory level in the quality of data. The types of data have to be kept as simple as possible for collection and processing, and the number of data items should be reduced to the barest minimum.

For these reasons, data from established sources frequently do not suffice for epidemiological purposes. With the developments in the methodology of epidemiological studies, *ad hoc* inquiries have been increasingly carried out in recent years in order to obtain data which are not covered by the established sources.

E

The epidemiologists' concern is not only restricted to the health status of the population *per se*. Many other facets of human life are relevant in epidemiological studies, such as education, economy, housing, labour conditions, delinquency, and meteorological conditions. Routine statistical data on these topics are available in a number of countries, but in this chapter discussions are limited mainly to the population, vital, and morbidity statistics.

Each country regularly publishes statistics compiled from established sources. In fact, numerous series of publications are issued in developed countries. Relevant national publications have to be consulted in the study of a particular topic, while for broad international comparisons it is convenient and useful to consult the United Nations *Demographic Yearbook* on population and vital statistics, and the World Health Organization *World Health Statistics Annual* on those of causes of death, morbidity, medical institutions, and health personnel. A monthly publication by the W.H.O., the *World Health Statistics Report*, presents statistics on specially chosen subjects as well as those on general current health. On statistics of widespread interest, the U.N. *Statistical Yearbook* is helpful.

POPULATION

Population statistics serve as background information for the planning and data analysis in epidemiological studies. The geographical distribution of the population and its composition with respect to age, sex, marital status, and economic characteristics are among the most useful basic data. They provide denominators, i.e. population at risk, in the calculation of mortality and morbidity rates.

Statistics derived from population censuses are available in most of the countries in the world. An effective mechanism for international co-ordination has been developed through the U.N. Principles and recommendations were formulated by the U.N. in consultation with individual countries in order to improve the census operations and the value of the compiled results for national purposes, and, wherever possible, to increase international comparability (U.N., 1967). In most countries a population census is undertaken once in every ten years, about the beginning of the decade, to collect demographic, economic, and social data on all persons in a country or in a well-delineated geographical area at a specified time. Priority items recommended by the U.N. (1967) are:

1. GEOGRAPHICAL CHARACTERISTICS

    i. place where found at time of census
    ii. place of birth

2. PERSONAL AND HOUSEHOLD CHARACTERISTICS
  i. sex
  ii. age
  iii. relationship to head of household
  iv. marital status
  v. children born alive
  vi. children living[1]
  vii. literacy[2]
  viii. school attendance[2]
  ix. educational attainment.

3. ECONOMIC CHARACTERISTICS
  i. type of activity (economically active or not)
  ii. occupation
  iii. industry
  iv. status (employer, employee, etc.)

Each country usually collects additional data, depending on its own requirements.

Certain data which do not require universal coverage are sometimes collected on a sample basis, for example from every tenth person or household visited by the enumerator. The scope of the census is then broadened at a small additional cost.

Population statistics by geographical subdivisions are compiled either according to the place where each person was found at the time of the census, or according to the place of usual residence. The two types of figures may show sizeable differences due to movements of seasonal workers and tourists. The epidemiological implication is that, in the computation of mortality and morbidity rates, an appropriate denominator should be used for population at risk.

Censuses are taken essentially for statistical purposes and special effort is made to reduce errors to a minimum. The figures collected in population censuses are therefore among the most reliable statistics obtained routinely.

Errors which occur include under- and overenumeration and errors in the content of each item. Infants are more likely to be omitted than persons at higher ages. Because the data on the newborn are unreliable, the age-specific rate is not usually calculated for age under 1 year. Instead the infant mortality rate is computed by using annual live births as the denominator.

---

[1] This applies primarily to countries where civil registration is either non-existent or deficient. Mortality rates can be estimated on the basis of this item and item v.

[2] These are for countries where literacy and school attendance do not involve the majority of the population.

In a population where birth registration is incomplete, the exact age of persons is often not ascertained. In these countries the age distribution reported in the census tends to be centred on certain numbers, such as those ending with '0' or '5'. For rating the accuracy of census age recording a system known as Whipple's Index is used, which indicates the degree of concentration of age reporting around '0' and '5' (U.N. *Demographic Yearbook*, 1955 and 1963).

In practice a census enumeration district is used as the unit area assigned to an enumerator or a small team of enumerators. Population data on each enumeration district are usually not published, but are available for use as a statistical 'frame' in the design of sample surveys which may be organized later on various topics, including health matters.

VITAL STATISTICS

Vital statistics are those statistics which are compiled on live births, deaths, foetal deaths, marriages, divorces, adoptions, legitimations, recognitions, annulments, and legal separations (U.N., 1953). In epidemiological studies the first three types of event have direct bearing, though marriages and divorces are also relevant in some studies.

In many countries vital statistics have been derived from civil registration developed primarily for legal purposes. In the U.N. *Demographic Yearbook* a registration system representing at least 90 per cent coverage of events is considered satisfactory; according to this criterion, only one-third of the world population is covered by civil registration with sufficient completeness.

There is, however, an acute need in each country for obtaining statistical data on fertility and mortality for use in national planning. To fulfil this need a number of sample surveys have been carried out in recent years in many developing countries in order to estimate the levels of fertility and mortality, without waiting for the full establishment of civil registration systems.

First priority items recommended by U.N. (1953) for statistical reports on live birth, death, foetal death, marriage, and divorce are as follows:

1. LIVE BIRTH

    i. *Characteristics of the event or child:*

        (*a*) attendant at birth
        (*b*) date of birth
        (*c*) date of registration
        (*d*) legitimacy
        (*e*) place of birth
        (*f*) sex
        (*g*) type of birth (i.e. single or plural)

ii. *Characteristics of mother:*

(*a*) date of birth (or age)
(*b*) number of children born to this mother
(*c*) place of usual residence

2. DEATH

i. *Characteristics of the event:*

(*a*) cause of death
(*b*) certifier
(*c*) date of death
(*d*) date of registration
(*e*) place of death

ii. *Characteristics of the deceased:*

(*a*) date of birth (or age)
(*b*) place of usual residence
(*c*) sex

3. FOETAL DEATH

i. *Characteristics of the event or product:*

(*a*) date of foetal delivery
(*b*) date of registration
(*c*) legitimacy
(*d*) period of gestation
(*e*) place of occurrence
(*f*) sex
(*g*) type of birth (i.e. single or plural)

ii. *Characteristics of the mother:*

(*a*) date of birth (or age)
(*b*) number of children born to this mother
(*c*) place of usual residence

4. MARRIAGE

i. *Characteristics of the event:*

(*a*) date of marriage
(*b*) place of marriage

ii. *Characteristics of the bride and groom:*

(*a*) date of birth (or age)
(*b*) marital status
(*c*) place of usual residence

5. DIVORCE

   i. *Characteristics of the event:*

     (*a*) date of divorce

     (*b*) place of divorce

  ii. *Characteristics of the divorcees:*

     (*a*) date of birth (or age)

     (*b*) date of marriage

     (*c*) number of dependent children

     (*d*) place of usual residence.

Other items are added depending upon each country's requirements. Items of epidemiological interest are, for birth reporting, the gestation period and birth weight, and for all five types of event, the socioeconomic characteristics.

When vital statistics are compiled by geographical subdivisions of a country, in principle they refer to the place of usual residence. However, statistics based on the place of occurrence are also compiled according to the needs of each country. The difference in the numbers may be considerable for birth and death, since many expectant mothers and sick persons move into large urban areas where more developed maternity services and medical care facilities are available. With some exceptions, such as deaths from traffic accidents and other acute conditions for which statistics by place of occurrence are relevant, vital events are more appropriately referred to the place of usual residence. Moreover, it may often be difficult to find the corresponding population at risk if rates are to be calculated by the place of occurrence.

In countries where a civil registration system exists the enforcement of registration is usually most strict for death, the burial being authorized only after the death is registered. Longer delays may occur in the registration of the other vital events.

Some under-registration may occur of deaths of the newborn, even in countries with nearly complete registration. Instead these deaths are likely to be reported as stillborn, causing omissions in the registration of live births and infant deaths. The effect of under-registration is proportionally more serious in the latter. It is for this reason that international comparability of the infant mortality rate is hampered. In many countries it is difficult to estimate the amount of bias, but as an example of a country with an excellent vital registration system, a recent report on infant mortality in the Netherlands states that the mortality of the first week of life is currently underestimated by 1·5 to 2 per 1,000 live births, which is about 10 per cent of the registered infant mortality rate (de Haas-Posthuma and de Haas, 1968).

TABLE 1 shows breakdowns of infant mortality by age for fifteen selected countries whose death registration is generally considered complete. The countries are arranged according to the post-neonatal mortality rate, i.e. for death at 28 days to under 1 year of age, which is likely to be accurate. The rates for 1 day or older generally follow the same sequence, but mortality under 1 day shows no regularity within the series. This is presumably caused by varying registration practice for deaths occurring soon after birth between different countries.

TABLE 1

INFANT MORTALITY RATE (PER 1,000 LIVE BIRTHS)
BY AGE IN SELECTED COUNTRIES 1965

COUNTRY	MORTALITY			
	Under 1 day	1–6 days	7–27 days	28 days to 11 months
Sweden	4·5	5·1	1·0	2·8
Australia	6·9	4·8	1·6	5·2
England and Wales . .	6·6	4·7	1·7	6·1
France	2·0	6·9	2·5	6·7
Japan	2·4	5·8	3·5	6·9
United States . . .	10·2	5·7	1·8	7·0
Czechoslovakia . . .	9·0	5·6	2·6	8·3
Singapore	4·6	9·4	3·8	8·4
Israel	5·4	6·9	3·3	11·6
Italy	8·6	8·5	5·2	13·7
Bulgaria	1·9	6·5	5·4	17·1
Mauritius ex. dep. . .	6·4	16·3	8·8	32·6
Mexico	2·8	11·5	8·6	37·8
Dominican Republic . .	2·3	10·9	12·5	47·0
Guatemala	7·2	12·0	16·0	57·4

Source: U.N. *Demographic Yearbook* 1967.

A concept of perinatal mortality, comprising both late-foetal and neonatal mortalities, was developed in order to cope, on one hand, with the above-mentioned difficulties in registration practice, and, on the other, with the fact that the underlying causes of both types of death have much in common. The definition frequently used refers to foetal deaths at 28 weeks of gestation or more and to deaths under 7 days, though the usage varies among countries. In most, the registration of late-foetal deaths is still incomplete and the degree of under-registration is therefore not known.

An item of great epidemiological importance in the study of deaths is the cause. Two indicators are used to judge broadly the degree of reliability of this information: first, the proportion of deaths certified by the physician attending the deceased during the last illness, and secondly, the proportion of deaths assigned to 'senility and ill-defined causes' (I.C.D. Code 790–6). For example, in most European countries more than 90 per cent of deaths are certified by physicians and the proportion of ill-defined causes does not exceed 10 per cent.

It does not follow, of course, that the cause of death well defined by a physician is always accurate. A study on 9,501 autopsies in selected hospitals in the United Kingdom by Heasman and Lipworth (1966) revealed that clinical and autopsy diagnoses agreed in only 45 per cent of the deaths, on the basis of the four-digit categories of the I.C.D. In another recent study conducted by the Pan American Health Organization on about 43,000 deaths in ten cities of Latin America and one city each in the United States and the United Kingdom, the original assignment of the cause of death was reviewed, together with all the available clinical, laboratory and pathological records, by two experienced referees in order to arrive at a final assignment of the cause. By using seventy-four groups of causes, 67 per cent of the original and final assignments agreed (Puffer and Wynne Griffith, 1967).

However, errors in classification occur in two different directions: some deaths from a particular cause are assigned wrongly to the other causes, while deaths from the other ones may be assigned wrongly to that cause. As statistics on the cause of death, if compiled routinely, do not involve much beyond frequency counts by age and sex, individual errors cancel each other out, at least partially, resulting in smaller net aggregate errors. In this sense the reliability of statistics on causes of death is higher than the individual accuracy would indicate. In fact, in both of the above-mentioned studies, in spite of the relatively large individual disagreement between original and final diagnoses, the total numbers of deaths assigned to a cause before and after review were frequently similar because of compensating differences, though important discrepancies still remained for several specific conditions.

Statistics on the cause of death from countries with incomplete death registration are generally unreliable, and even sample surveys provide no better information because they are usually based on retrospective inquiries.

Death certificates are processed in national vital statistics offices by coding the underlying cause of death. The suitability and usefulness of the concept of the underlying cause of death have been questioned in recent years, especially by workers in developed countries where the majority of deaths occur at advanced age and involve several serious pathological conditions simultaneously. So far, tabulations of national data on a multiple cause basis have not been feasible, because of the large amount of coding required and the complications in the tabulation procedure. However, now that computer facilities are more widely available studies of multiple cause analysis are progressing in Europe and North America.

Some caution is needed when the registered marriage rate is used for epidemiological study, because national practice of registration varies. In a population where advantages of legal entitlements of marriage are not considered important, a considerable degree of under-registration and long delays in registration may occur, so much so that the rates derived will be of little scientific value.

There are a number of sources from which morbidity statistics are compiled routinely. At least some kind of morbidity statistics is, in fact, available in almost every country of the world.

Two sources which are most frequently available for the compilation of routine morbidity statistics are notification of disease and hospital in-patient records. Moreover, statistics are compiled from records at other medical care services in a number of countries. In developed countries social security records provide an additional source of information on the amount of morbidity in the population covered by the system.

Statistics from Notification and Registration of Diseases

In the strict sense of the word, 'notification' means a mere reporting of the occurrence of an event, while 'registration' denotes the legal recording with the authorized officials of the occurrence of an event (U.N., 1953). To some extent, however, the two words are loosely used in the reporting of disease occurrence. A major distinction in the purpose of reporting is that notification serves to enable health authorities to initiate an immediate action to control the spread of the disease while registration serves more for the follow-up of patients.

The International Sanitary Regulations stipulate that the member countries of the W.H.O. should report the incidence of quarantinable diseases (smallpox, cholera, plague, yellow fever, typhus, and relapsing fever) to the W.H.O., which in turn should disseminate the information to all member countries. In addition to these, each country has a list of other notifiable diseases which are of public health importance to the country. The list contains mostly acute communicable diseases, though in some industrialized countries certain occupational diseases are also notifiable. Information collected by the W.H.O. on the national notification practice on thirty-six selected conditions was studied by Taylor (1965).

Individual records collected cover age, sex, and date and place of occurrence of disease. Other items such as occupation, first symptoms, laboratory confirmation, and previous vaccinations are included in some countries.

Since the primary purpose of notification is to warn the health authorities of the danger of a possible epidemic, suspected cases are also notified at once, though later reports may provide information on the confirmation of suspected cases. In the first case the reported figures need not be, and in fact are far from, accurate enough for elaborate analysis. The completeness of reporting depends on the conditions of each country, and varies according to the disease and also chronologically. For example, Lossing (1955) reported that notification of measles, whooping cough, chickenpox, mumps, and German measles in Canada covered only10–17 per cent of the total incidence of these diseases. According to a British study by Stocks (1949) diseases such as diphtheria and scarlet fever were fairly completely notified, measles was reported for 66 per cent but whooping cough only about 20 per cent. The difference between the two countries was caused presumably by the existence of a national health insurance scheme in the United Kingdom where physicians are encouraged more to report the disease incidence.

The reliability of statistics on notifiable diseases is generally so low, and international comparability so poor, that the data may seem almost useless for study of the magnitude of the incidence. Nevertheless, where no sudden changes are suspected in the coverage and content, the figures collected from notifications within a country can be used for certain analysis such as the study of epidemic curves and geographical propagation of an epidemic, as well as analysis of trends. A few suggestions were made by a W.H.O. Expert Committee for improving the completeness and representativeness of the reporting of notifiable diseases. Since the longer the list of notifiable diseases the less likely it is that reporting will be complete, a periodic review was particularly recommended so as to keep in the list only those strictly relevant to the disease problem of the localities, regions, or countries concerned (W.H.O., 1968).

Registration systems have been instituted in a number of countries for patients suffering from certain chronic diseases of great social importance. Leprosy patients are now registered in most countries where the disease is endemic. A tuberculosis register is also in operation in a number of countries, while in recent years registration of cancer and congenital disorders has been started in developed countries. If a complete register is maintained in good order, current information should, theoretically, be available on incidence, prevalence, case fatality and recovery rates, together with associated factors. The completeness of coverage varies from country to country, depending on the efficiency in case detection. Multiple registration may also be necessary for the same patients, unless a central national registry exists. However, the epidemiological value of statistics from registries is limited at present since reliable follow-up data, especially the outcome of medical care, are often not available.

Morbidity Statistics from Medical Care Services

Hospital in-patient statistics are available in a great number of countries. These statistics usually cover hospitals run by the government authorities, but private hospitals are often included too. The statistics are based on medical records kept on individual patients and in most cases are compiled from information available at the time of discharge. As their primary objective, in-patient statistics give useful information for the planning of hospital services. In comparison with morbidity statistics from the other established sources, hospital statistics are supported by diagnostic data far more accurate than is possible elsewhere. In spite of this advantage, their value in the study of general morbidity is seriously limited for two reasons:

1. The catchment population is usually unknown and consequently population-based rates cannot be computed.
2. The types of disease represented in hospital statistics are highly selective, influenced by the local availability of hospital services, the policy of hospitalization, and the habit of the population.

Minimum requirements on tabulations recommended by a W.H.O. Expert Committee included tables on the annual number of discharges and duration of hospitalization, according to diagnosis and sex. The use of the I.C.D. was recommended for the classification of diagnosis (W.H.O., 1963).

Statistics are also published on patients at specialized hospitals and sanatoria, and the specialized departments of general hospitals. Services for mental disorder, tuberculosis, leprosy, and maternity are covered by many countries, while in some developed ones statistical reports are issued on patients in cancer and paediatric hospitals.

Regular reports published by individual countries often cover morbidity data collected from out-patient services of hospitals, clinics, health centres, and general practitioners. There is much less uniformity in the recording procedures and, consequently, completeness and quality of diagnosis and other data in published statistics are mostly questionable. *Ad hoc* inquiries by sampling are undertaken in some countries in order to extract useful data from this source on specially designed record forms.

Morbidity Statistics from Social Security Systems

With the rapid growth of social security systems in more developed countries in recent decades, new series of reports are now published on statistics compiled from insurance claims and records of industrial absenteeism. The population at risk is, in principle, well defined and hence appropriate morbidity rates can be worked out. The data are of particular value when the whole population of a community or a country is covered by the system. The files in a large-scale social security system are, however, usually decentralized and the statistical processing of records is not necessarily well organized. The types of morbidity covered and the representativeness of the records depends so much on the particular conditions of each system that a careful study is needed on the use of the derived statistics.

DATA ON DRUG QUESTIONS

The thalidomide accidents in recent years gave a spurt for developed countries to organize a drug monitoring scheme. Animal experiments and clinical trials on man, which are usually limited in size and scope, cannot predict many of the adverse reactions which occur infrequently or which have varied effects on different populations according to their age, sex, and pathology. The primary object of drug monitoring is, therefore, to detect the capacity of a drug to produce undesirable effects at the earliest time possible after it is put on to the market (W.H.O., 1966).

A number of countries are developing a national system in which adverse reactions of drugs are reported by practising physicians and hospitals to monitoring centres. At present the coverage in most monitoring systems does not yet reach 10 per cent of all the reactions which occur in the country.

For reactions which are rare or which differ in their frequency and severity depending on genetic, climatic (e.g. amount of sunlight), and other conditions affecting the population, consolidation of data from different countries will be of considerable value. For this purpose an international monitoring system is being developed by the W.H.O. Priority items of data collected include age and sex of patient, drug names (suspected and others), dosage regime, and description of adverse reactions.

Analysis carried out regularly on these reports should identify suspected drugs. However, a more detailed epidemiological study is required in each instance for establishing a causal relationship, since data from a monitoring system, as they are currently collected, do not provide suitable figures for the population at risk and, moreover, no control groups are readily available for comparison of the incidence of the suspected adverse effect ascribed to a particular drug. In general, further research is needed on the methodology of efficient routine analysis of data.

FUTURE PROSPECTS

Developments in routine data collection are envisaged in three directions, namely:

1. Improvement in the coverage and accuracy of data from traditional sources.

2. Greater flexibility in the storage and retrieval of data.

3. Establishment of new routine sources to cope with changing health needs.

Constant efforts are being made to improve the currently available routine data collection schemes, both by national authorities and international agencies. In developing countries the need for complete civil registration and improved morbidity reporting systems will be increasingly recognized. Such developments will, however, be a slow process which depends on the progress in the basic health services of a country and more generally on the improvements in the general level of living.

Use of computers is revolutionizing the data handling in every branch of science. One of the advantages of automatic devices is an increased flexibility in the use of data. Moreover, storage, retrieval, and linkage of various sources of data are greatly facilitated by the use of computers. In order to reduce human intervention in data handling to a minimum, the record forms need to be redesigned for automatic processing, for example to make them suitable for automatic document readers which are used in an increasing number of developed countries.

A remarkable progress is envisaged in more developed countries in the routine collection of morbidity data. Medical record systems are now undergoing rapid changes so that voluminous data on individual patients may be stored and information from various sources merged together in a computer-based file. Information on individuals can then be retrieved at any time to help physicians to provide the patients with appropriate medical care. A carefully organized computer file should enable epidemiologists and health administrators to obtain useful statistical tabulations both on a routine and on an *ad hoc* basis.

REFERENCES

DE HAAS-POSTHUMA, J. H., and DE HAAS, J. H. (1968) *Infant Loss in the Netherlands*, National Center for Health Statistics, Series 3, No. 11, Public Health Service, United States Department of Health, Education and Welfare, Washington, D.C.

HEASMAN, M. A., and LIPWORTH, L. (1966) *Accuracy of Certification of Cause of Death*, Studies on Medical and Population Subjects, No. 20, General Register Office, London, H.M.S.O.

LOSSING, E. G. (1955) Reporting of notifiable diseases, *Canad. J. publ. Hlth*, **46**, 444.

PUFFER, R. R., and WYNNE GRIFFITH, G. (1967) *Patterns of Urban Mortality*, Scientific Publication No. 151, Pan American Health Organization, Washington, D.C.

STOCKS, P. (1949) *Sickness and the Population of England and Wales*, Studies on Medical and Population Subjects, No. 2, General Register Office, London, H.M.S.O.

TAYLOR, I. (1965) The notification of infectious diseases in various countries, in *Trends in the Study of Morbidity and Mortality*, Public Health Papers, No. 27, World Health Organization, Geneva.

UNITED NATIONS (1953) *Principles for a Vital Statistics System. Recommendations for the Improvement and Standardisation of Vital Statistics*, Statistical Papers, Series M., No. 19, Statistical Office of the U.N., New York.

UNITED NATIONS (1967) *Principles and Recommendations for the 1970 Population Censuses*, Statistical Papers, Series M., No. 44, Statistical Office of the U.N., New York.

WORLD HEALTH ORGANIZATION (1963) Eighth Report of the Expert Committee on Health Statistics, Technical Report Series No. 261, Geneva.

WORLD HEALTH ORGANIZATION (1966) *International Monitoring of Adverse Reactions to Drugs*, Official Records of the W.H.O., No. 148, Annex 11, Geneva.

WORLD HEALTH ORGANIZATION (1968) *Morbidity Statistics*, Twelfth Report of the Expert Committee on Health Statistics, Technical Report Series No. 389, Geneva.

6

SURVEY TECHNIQUES

W. E. WATERS AND P. C. ELWOOD

QUESTIONNAIRE DESIGN

GENERAL CONSIDERATIONS

'No survey is better than its questionnaire.' The design of a questionnaire should be one of the main considerations in planning a survey. Once a hypothesis has been formulated, it is often useful to sketch out in some detail the tables which will have to be constructed to enable the hypothesis to be tested. Only when this has been done should the questionnaire be completed to provide the answers to obtain the data for the tables. Such an approach will greatly facilitate decisions on the relevance of particular questions, and will help to avoid the collection of irrelevant and ambiguous data.

There are two kinds of questionnaire: those which are self-administered, that is, completed by the subject, and those which are completed by an interviewer. Most of what will be said here is relevant to both, though many of the points apply with greater force to the self-administered form. In general, this form is better, as one important source of bias, the interviewer, is avoided. On the other hand, a questionnaire which is to be completed by a subject must be relatively short and simple, while one which is administered can be longer and of considerable complexity. A compromise approach is sometimes possible in which a self-administered questionnaire is filled up by a subject under the supervision of an interviewer who can, if necessary, give a limited amount of help.

The problem of bias has been mentioned above and a few general considerations of its nature are now given, as bias is one of the greatest problems in medical research. One must continually have it in mind to reduce its effects, and to prevent oneself drawing erroneous conclusions. Used in this context bias may be defined as any unwanted or unplanned interaction. However meticulous the investigation, errors or variations are bound to occur in any measurements. If these errors are of a random type, they are less of a problem than if they are of the constant systematic type which are the sources of bias. Examples of bias in questionnaires are given later in this chapter.

Questionnaires should be simply and clearly laid out. This applies both to the general design and to the individual questions. It also applies to instructions on the questionnaire. For example, many a questionnaire has been ruined because the method of answering questions has not been clearly stated and illustrated, and it may be impossible to score questionnaires when some of the answers have been ringed, and others have been crossed out or underlined.

Confidentiality should be assured in any medical study. This may be achieved by a simple statement printed clearly at the top of each form, and it should be reinforced by being read out if the questionnaire is administered.

If any part is played by an interviewer, it is most important that this is carefully rehearsed and standardized, otherwise considerable bias may be introduced. This applies even if a questionnaire is handed to subjects on a doorstep or on leaving a clinic. The invitation to complete and return it, together with any instructions must be given in exactly the same way, and even in the same tone of voice, to each subject. If a questionnaire is administered, bias will probably be introduced, and if several interviewers are used the direction and degree of bias may be different for each. It is advisable, therefore, to use a single interviewer, or, if this is not possible, it is best if subjects are allocated to different interviewers at random so that bias from this source will be balanced within subgroups of the population surveyed.

The first consideration in designing a questionnaire is to make it clear and unambiguous to the person who has to fill it in. This should never be compromised, even if it is to be administered by a trained interviewer. However, detailed thought should also be given at an early stage to coding. Sometimes a punch card can be prepared directly from the questionnaire and, though this may not always be possible, it should seldom be necessary to transcribe information on to an intermediate coding sheet. Such a process is wasteful and increases the likelihood of errors. Simple measures such as keeping the answers to the right-hand margin, always coding 'No' as '0', etc., can save a lot of time and temper subsequently. Another simple aid is to put all data which will be used to classify the population in one place, so that bundles of questionnaires can be quickly sorted into subgroups defined by, for example, age and sex. Special boxes for coding can be printed on the questionnaires but care must be taken to prevent subjects writing their answers in these spaces.

FRAMING THE QUESTIONS

Framing questions in an interview, whether this is scripted or spontaneous, is an art. It is essential from the start to have a clear idea of what is wanted from the interview, and individual questions should be constructed so as to give the exact data, and only that data, necessary to achieve the aim of the study. One should therefore re-examine a questionnaire repeatedly during its preparation, and eliminate any questions which are not of direct relevance.

There are numerous important considerations in wording a question. Certain words or phrases may have different meanings in different areas, and a slight change in wording, or in the context in which a question is asked, may markedly affect the response. However, it is difficult to derive principles which will be of value in every relevant situation. During the testing of a questionnaire—and this should not be confined to discussions with colleagues—many of the ambiguous and imprecise questions will be detected. However, many of the unsatisfactory aspects of a questionnaire may not become evident until it is used in the field, and a small pilot survey is therefore essential in most, if not all, studies. A pilot study loses much of its point if it is not conducted in a sample of subjects reasonably representative of the population of interest.

Although questionnaires, especially of the self-administered form, should have less bias than conventional clinical interviews, this can rarely be completely eliminated. There are personality differences between subjects and some are always more willing to answer 'Yes' than others, irrespective of the questions asked. Similarly, some individuals tend always to give extreme responses on rating-scales, again irrespective of the specific quality that they are asked to rate (Ingham, 1969). These tendencies are likely to be affected by cultural influences and in comparisons between communities they may be confused with differences in the prevalence of illnesses (Epstein, 1969).

Another form of bias is prompted by the situation in which the questionnaire is completed. For example a patient who attends a doctor for treatment is more inclined to answer 'Yes' to almost any question relevant to his or her health, while a subject who has been asked, or perhaps persuaded, to co-operate in a survey is more likely to answer 'No' to the same questions. The subject's motivation may also be important: Heron (1956) found, for example, that when a questionnaire was given to applicants for a job the 'neurotic' responses differed depending on whether the subjects thought the questions part of the selection procedure or for research purposes.

There are ways of avoiding bias to some extent. One which we have found very useful is to present a series of statements about a symptom and ask the subject to choose the one which is nearest to the truth. If the statements used in this method are chosen to represent different severities of a system, this method also gives a crude grade. The statements can be presented in a logical manner, for example as a series representing increasing severities or frequencies, or the order can be randomized. For example, several answers can be suggested for a question, each one implying a different frequency:

F

$$
\text{Do you get a headache?} \left\{
\begin{array}{ll}
\text{— never} & \text{Grade (1)} \\
\text{— seldom} & (2) \\
\text{— occasionally} & (3) \\
\text{— frequently} & (4) \\
\text{— very often} & (5)
\end{array}
\right.
$$

A much more sophisticated method of presenting such statements is described for administered questionnaires by Ingham (1965) and for the self-administered form by Wood and Elwood (1966).

TESTING THE QUESTIONNAIRE

Although the initial design of a questionnaire is largely an art, the testing should be both rigorous and scientific. An ideal questionnaire should be acceptable, reproducible, sensitive, and specific. However, it is seldom possible to confirm the presence of all these desirable characteristics in a questionnaire before it is applied in large-scale surveys. Indeed, testing on a considerable scale may well be required to fully establish any one of these characteristics.

Acceptability is not usually a problem in medical questionnaires. The reasons for doing the survey should be briefly outlined, and the relevance of each question should, if possible, be obvious, otherwise some further explanation should be given. For example, questions about employment, the answers to which will be used to classify a population by social class, usually seem irrelevant in a medical context. Obviously, questions should be worded so that they do not offend, and it may occasionally be necessary to consider whether or not a question will worry a patient or precipitate neurosis. On occasions we have buried within a questionnaire a series of questions, whose answers enabled a crude 'neurotic grade' to be derived for the respondent. This grading had previously been shown to correlate fairly closely with a psychiatrist's opinion. However, the questions, if presented together, were too obviously psychiatric in content to be acceptable in a general health questionnaire, though scattered through a longer questionnaire they seemed not to be regarded as unusual. Although using the questions in this way undoubtedly altered the pattern of responses they did enable valid comparisons between subgroups to be made. Acceptability of a questionnaire may also be affected by length and place of origin, and Cartwright and Ward (1968) have presented evidence that in a postal survey a short questionnaire posted locally elicits the best response rate. Thus, with postal questionnaires, one must compromise between the likely response rate and the amount of information that one is able to collect.

To be useful and meaningful, measurements must be reasonably reproducible. That is, there should be good agreement between repeated measurements, provided all other relevant variables (such as diurnal variation) are controlled. Fundamentally, reproducibility is the sum of subject variation and observer variation. With a self-administered questionnaire the subject and observer variation are really combined, but in administered questionnaires both subject and observer variation are present separately, and both may be very important. Variation on the part of the observer can be easily demonstrated, as even questions which are phrased in an identical manner may elicit different answers with different interviewers when questioning random samples of a single population. Variation on the part of the subjects is more difficult to examine. The same questionnaire cannot be put to the same individuals after the lapse of only a short interval of time, and if a long period is allowed to elapse between interviews any difference in response may be due either to real changes with time or to subject variation. However, certain aspects of subject variation can sometimes be examined by asking the same or similar questions in different parts of a questionnaire, which will reveal any inconsistent responses. Such a technique may occasionally be detected by a subject and cause irritation, but some warning of this can be given beforehand by telling the subject that an attempt is being made to assess the best method of obtaining certain items of information. We have found that a higher proportion of subjects said that they had been free of headaches in the previous year, when the relevant questions were presented as part of a general health survey, than when the questions formed part of a questionnaire concerned entirely with headache. Many such instances probably occur and the need for standardization in all aspects of collecting data for research cannot be stressed too strongly or too often. This is particularly important if a questionnaire is to be used for comparison between different areas, but unfortunately complete standardization for such studies is difficult and often impossible. In such circumstances it may be important to quantify differences which occur when the questionnaire is used in different languages. Such differences should be sought by applying the questionnaire in one or more ways, each method being carried out on a random sample of the same population.

An attempt must be made to 'validate' a questionnaire. Until this is done it is simply a list of questions and one can only assume that it is measuring something that is meaningful in clinical terms. The validity of a questionnaire is the extent to which it gives a true assessment of what it is intended to measure, and to test this some independent, and preferably objective, test is required. Thus the validity of the London School of Hygiene and Tropical Medicine questionnaire on anginal chest pain has been assessed by comparing estimates of the prevalence of coronary artery disease based on its use alone, on an unscripted clinical interview, on electrocardiographic findings, and on follow-up studies (Rose, 1965). With conditions that are sometimes fatal an examination of the subsequent mortality experience of subjects, in relation to their answers to various questions, may be one of the most useful tests of the value of a questionnaire. In fact, validity depends both on 'sensitivity' and 'specificity'. Sensitivity is simply the proportion of the subjects affected by a condition which is identified by any particular diagnostic method. The more sensitive the method the smaller the proportion of affected subjects which is missed—that is, the number of 'false negatives' is low. A diagnostic method is specific if it does not include subjects other than those with the condition in which one is interested, that is, there are few 'false positives'. Obviously one cannot expect a questionnaire to give no false positives and no false negatives. The ratio between false positives and false negatives which is acceptable for any particular study will depend on many circumstances. In population screening it is usually more important to avoid false negatives, that is, to avoid missing cases, than to include a number of false positives as these can usually be eliminated at a later stage by further confirmatory tests. However, the additional testing of large numbers of individuals is wasteful and may cause anxiety. It can also harm the response to a large community survey if it becomes realized that co-operation leads to further investigations for many of those that attend.

THE SURVEY
PLANNING THE SURVEY

Surveys may be broadly thought of as of two kinds. In observational surveys one is trying to get an estimate of certain population parameters such as the age distribution, or the proportion with bronchitis or ischaemic heart disease, etc. The other main type of survey is that in which one is testing a hypothesis. Examples of suitable hypotheses are numerous in the literature, for instance, the hypothesis that tobacco smoking and symptoms of chronic bronchitis are associated, or that ischaemic heart disease is related to serum lipids or sugar intake in the diet.

The objectives of a survey must be clearly defined at an early stage. A casual 'look-see' attitude usually leads to nothing but confusion, and the use of data collected during a study to test a hypothesis which is formulated after the event, may invalidate the conventional methods of testing statistical significance. When a survey is being designed it is not enough to state only the general aims, for example, to study the nutritional status of elderly people. The objectives must be listed in more precise terms, that is—to use the same example—to determine, in a representative sample of subjects of both sexes aged 65 years and over, the distributions of height, weight, skinfold thickness, circulating haemoglobin, serum folate and B_{12}, and leucocyte ascorbic acid. The most efficient surveys are probably those in which one or more hypotheses are tested, while at the same time observational data are collected which are required to formulate any further hypotheses. For example, in a survey such as the one just mentioned estimates of blood urea level might be obtained in each subject to facilitate the designing of subsequent studies of renal function in elderly subjects. Such a technique ensures the continuous employment of the epidemiologist and his staff.

The practical design of any study depends on its objectives, and only when those have been clearly formulated can one proceed. The next step is to sketch out the statistical tables, etc., which will be required to test any given hypothesis before designing the study that will give the data for these tables. Such a technique will not only indicate the nature of these data, but will also assist in the estimation of the size of the sample required. It will also become clear in most studies which data can be collected during the initial survey, which need only be collected from a subsample of the population surveyed, and which can only be efficiently collected during a follow-up study of subjects identified during the initial survey. In the example given above, one might collect data relating to body measurements from all the subjects surveyed, but take a blood sample from only a random third of the subjects seen, and perhaps return and conduct a detailed dietary study on only those found to have low levels of serum folate, etc.

Once a design has been decided for a study this should be fully outlined in a document, which in turn should be circulated widely for comments. Specialists in different fields should be contacted: in the project outlined above epidemiologists, statisticians, geriatricians, clinicians, haematologists, biochemists, nutritionists, dieticians and welfare officers of the local authority may all have useful and relevant points of view. One must guard against the danger, however, of incorporating too many inquiries in a study; too many of the experts approached may feel that their most useful comments will relate to further items which could be added to the inquiry. The ethical aspects of all research should be discussed fully with colleagues, and if necessary referred to independent observers.

Drawing the sample for a study is one of the most important steps. However, detailed discussion of all the relevant considerations is inappropriate here, and decisions can only be made when the objectives have been formulated. Unfortunately other considerations, such as the resources and skills available, usually need to be taken into account also. At this stage one should come to a decision about non-responders; it is all too easy to make biased decisions at the end of a study about which of the non-responders can be excluded. Numerous reasons for non-response will arise during a study— some will clearly be outside the criteria of the study by reasons of age or area of normal residence, while others may be unsuitable by reason of illness, senility, mental deficiency, blindness, etc., but they are not necessarily outside the criteria of the study and exclusion of such subjects may be inappropriate. Refusal to co-operate on the part of some subjects is a problem in all surveys. The size of this proportion in a sample can be minimized by refining the initial approach to subjects, by making repeated requests for co-operation and perhaps enlisting the help of the family doctor. Non-response, however, seldom completely invalidates conclusions of a study. One may afterwards be able to estimate the effect of non-response on the data, particularly if some data, such as age and sex, are available for those who are not included.

The planning stage of the survey will include the selection of suitable questionnaires or the design of new ones. These problems have been discussed above. All other tests (e.g. blood tests, X-rays, electrocardiograms, pulmonary function tests, etc.) should be reviewed in a similar manner and their acceptability, reproducibility, sensitivity and specificity ascertained. The effects of any observer and diurnal or seasonal variation should be reviewed, and as far as possible any bias that these may produce should be kept to a minimum by the design of the survey. A review of the medical literature during the planning stage will help provide information on many of these aspects. This information is often widely scattered, but for cardiovascular surveys the World Health Organization monograph by Rose and Blackburn (1968) is a model of helpfulness.

FIELD SURVEY ORGANIZATION

When the details of the information to be collected by the survey have been decided, the practical aspects of organization must be considered. These include the method of contacting the subjects in the survey sample and consultations about the survey with other interested people. These arrangements obviously differ according to the nature of the survey and how the subjects are selected. At the Medical Research Council Epidemiology Unit (South Wales) subjects are usually selected from Electoral Rolls or after a private census of a defined area. It is usually found that direct contact by a specially trained home visitor, calling at the subject's house, sometimes after a preliminary letter, is the best method of obtaining a high response rate. Alternatively, subjects may be sent letters by post outlining the purpose of the survey and what is required of them; or if they have a telephone this is another possible method of contact. However, we believe that a personal approach is usually better; one of the disadvantages of both the postal and telephone methods is that it is easier for the subjects to refuse to co-operate. Once a subject has refused, any subsequent contact is much more difficult, as few people like others to see that they have changed their minds on such an issue. One of the skills of a good home visitor is to be so friendly that subjects do not like to give a firm negative reply—if the visitor encounters any resistance the subject can be given a very brief outline of the survey and told to think it over. When contacted again a few days later the subject may have changed his attitude completely and may then be very co-operative. Such a change will be helped if he hears favourable reports of the survey from neighbours who have already participated. In many cases however, there is no apparent reason for this change.

Before any survey starts it is important for other interested organizations and individuals to be fully informed of the proposals. Thus the general practitioners and Medical Officers of Health in the survey area should be contacted either personally or by letter, or preferably by both methods. This is not only sound etiquette; their co-operation at a later stage may help towards the success of this survey and any subsequent one. It is not uncommon for individuals asked to co-operate in a medical survey to discuss it with their own doctor, and his attitude is obviously likely to be more helpful if he is fully aware at an early stage of what is being done in the survey. It may also be wise to inform the police that a medical survey is being conducted in their area, and possibly representatives of employers' organizations and trade union officials too. In surveys including minors, parental consent may be advisable.

It is usually a good thing to run the survey at a central 'clinic' or in a series of 'clinics'. These may be existing public health clinics or the surgeries of general practitioners. When these are not available, however, a school or church hall often provides an adequate centre, and a list of buildings that have been used by the Epidemiology Unit might surprise a hospital-based doctor! It is the usual policy of the Unit to provide cars to bring subjects to the clinic and drive them home after they have been seen. This service not only encourages them to attend but makes appointment systems more efficient by considerably reducing the number of booked appointments which are not filled. Subjects coming in 'under their own steam' are more likely to lapse, and skilled medical and technicians' time may be wasted. Furthermore, the use of transport and appointments reduces the subjects' waiting time at the centre and a well-run survey helps to increase the response rate.

Alternatively, subjects may be seen in their own homes. Such domiciliary visiting usually produces a higher response rate as the very busy, and those confined to home for any reason, can then be seen. Moreover, nervous subjects, who refuse to attend a clinic, may agree to the same tests being carried out in their own homes. On the other hand, domiciliary visits are usually more time-consuming for the survey team and this is particularly so if special investigations such as X-rays or electrocardiographs are being taken. Another important point is that the quality of the results obtained by portable equipment may be considerably inferior to that obtained at a clinic. Often the survey will compromise, with some people seen at central clinics and the remainder visited in their homes. In these cases it is important to consider to what extent bias may be introduced into the results.

At the beginning of the survey a definite plan for dealing with the results must be prepared. Who is told what, will depend very much both on the nature of the survey and on the personal views of the survey team. Sometimes, each subject can be given his results either at the time of the survey or later. On the other hand, many individuals express the view that they do not wish to know if anything is wrong. If no effective medical treatment is available for the abnormality found, this attitude has much to recommend in it. It is often convenient to tell subjects that they will only be contacted again if anything is found that requires 'further investigation or treatment'. This avoids the problem of deciding whether each individual result is normal or abnormal (never an easy task, since most surveys measure continuous variables). This method also avoids the possibility of producing unnecessary worry, or even a neurosis, by informing subjects of abnormal results of which they were previously unaware. The nature of the report is often ill understood, and no treatment may be necessary.

As a general rule the subject's doctor should be informed of all abnormal findings and a course of action for cases found during the survey should be arranged before the survey starts. Sometimes, doctors in the survey team may themselves deal with such treatment, but always after consultation with the subject's own doctor. At other times, cases may be referred to the local hospital out-patients' department or to specialized clinics—arrangements for the number of cases likely to be found should already have been made. The survey team can arrange these appointments and may provide help with transport for the cases. Rather surprisingly, the finding of cases and the prompt and efficient organizing of specialized investigations and treatment do not necessarily help the general image of the survey in the area being studied. Indeed neighbours of such cases are apt to see a 'cause and effect' sequence and blame the individual's admission to hospital on his attendance at the survey! It is important that the team help such individuals and their families as much as possible, particularly by making sure that they fully understand what is happening and why. There is often a sudden change from what is primarily a research project to the therapeutic management of individual patients. Such individuals often differ from other patients in that they did not seek medical help but were simply persuaded to help in a medical survey. In return, they should receive every consideration from the survey team, who bear responsibility for seeing that they are offered any necessary investigation or treatment.

Most of the practical aspects of survey organization described above are the results of experience in the field. They do not necessarily describe the only methods of conducting surveys. We are aware that experience, and success, with one particular method can all too easily lead to the belief that it is the only method. Yet there is no reason why the same scientific methods that lie behind the surveys should not be used to investigate the organization of the survey itself. While such ways of investigating survey methods may be time-consuming at first they may later make the running of surveys more efficient. Thus when two possible methods of conducting a survey are being debated they should be randomized to see which is, in fact, the better. During a haematological survey we conducted recently there was a difference of opinion as to whether or not direct mention of a blood test should be made in the initial letter sent to the subjects. The letters were therefore randomized —one half made specific mention of a blood test while the other made no special mention of this, but was otherwise identical. The results showed a slightly, though not significantly, higher response rate in the case of those letters specifically mentioning the blood test. Such randomized controlled trials of survey methods should be used whenever possible to inject a more scientific approach into the art of running surveys.

CROSS-SECTIONAL AND LONGITUDINAL STUDIES

Before a survey starts it will have been considered whether it is to be a single cross-sectional survey or whether a follow-up over a period of time will markedly increase the amount of information obtained. In general, cross-sectional studies provide data on prevalence rates, but the incidence (or attack) rates require measurements in the same individuals at more than one point in time. When considering aetiological hypotheses, longitudinal studies enable this to be done prospectively and thus avoid many of the biases inherent in retrospective studies.

If a longitudinal study is contemplated this may affect decisions on the best population to survey; consideration should therefore be given to the likely trend of migration of subjects from the survey area. Subjects can be told that the tests may be repeated in a few years' time. Our own experience has been that requests for subjects to notify changes of address are not a completely satisfactory way of keeping track of the sample. It may, however, be possible to record some individual identity number for each subject, which may enable them to be traced centrally. Even if subjects are not seen again, a limited follow-up may be undertaken after a period of years to determine the mortality experience of the various subgroups identified during the cross-sectional survey. The subsequent mortality experience is one of the most practical 'validations' of the original data, both that obtained by questionnaire and that obtained by other investigations such as haematological and biochemical tests, X-ray, ECGs, etc. This mortality information adds greatly to the value of the original observations.

REFERENCES

CARTWRIGHT, A., and WARD, A. W. M. (1968) Variations in general practitioners' response to postal questionnaires, *Brit. J. prev. soc. Med.*, **22**, 212.

EPSTEIN, L. M. (1969) Validity of a questionnaire for diagnosis of peptic ulcer in an ethnically heterogeneous population, *J. chron. Dis.*, **22**, 49.

HERON, A. (1956) The effects of real-life motivation on questionnaire response, *J. appl. Psychol.*, **40**, 65.

INGHAM, J. G. (1965) A method for observing symptoms and attitudes, *Brit. J. soc. clin. Psychol.*, **4**, 131.

INGHAM, J. G. (1969) Quantitative evaluation of subjective symptoms, *Proc. roy. Soc. Med.*, **62**, 492.

ROSE, G. A. (1965) Ischaemic heart disease. Chest pain questionnaire, *Milbank mem. Fd Quart.*, **43(2)**, 32.

ROSE, G. A., and BLACKBURN, H. (1968) Cardiovascular survey methods, *Wld Hlth Org. Monogr. Ser.*, No. 56.

WOOD, M. M., and ELWOOD, P. C. (1966) Symptoms of iron deficiency anaemia. A community survey, *Brit. J. prev. soc. Med.*, **20**, 117.

PART IV

RECORD LINKAGE

7

USES OF RECORD LINKAGE IN EPIDEMIOLOGY

M. A. HEASMAN

INTRODUCTION

RECORD linkage is the process of bringing together data recorded at different times and places into a series of personal cumulative files (Acheson, 1967; Preface, p. xvii[1]). There is nothing new in the concept; it has been used for a number of years by scientific workers in many fields. Typical examples of these are Doll and Bradford Hill (1964), who linked the death certificates of doctors with previously recorded smoking histories, and Stewart, Webb, and Hewitt (1958), who linked hospital records, birth, and death certificates in their survey of childhood malignancies. In the days before computers came into general use, the only means of linkage available to the research worker who wanted to create a linked file was to collect data laboriously from different sources in every way available to him. Each study involved an immense effort, and consequently it had to be very seriously considered whether the result was likely to repay this effort. How many worthwhile studies were never started for this reason will never be known.

The position at the time of writing (1969) is regrettably not very different but thanks to the pioneering work of Newcombe (1965) and Acheson (1967, 1968) it is now beginning to change. Within a very few years there should be several countries able to provide record linkage files in the medical field on a national basis.

By bringing together in one file summary records of medical and vital events, as a part of the routine processing of these records for statistical and other analyses, a whole new field of research is opened up. This is not so much because new information is available, but because information previously difficult to obtain as it was held in files widely separated from each other becomes so much more easily accessible. The speed of the computer and the rapidity with which it can process material not only opens up new vistas for the research worker but develops a potential of great value to clinicians and administrators.

[1] The book by E. D. Acheson, *Medical Record Linkage*, and a second edited by him (1968) should be consulted by all who wish to know more about the possibilities and methods of record linkage.

This chapter does not deal with the methods of record linkage. It is not a subject with which the average epidemiologist needs to be excessively familiar, any more than he needs to know much about the internal working of a computer. Neither is it a subject which is exclusively of medical interest. Record linkage is being developed in fields of education, social administration, etc., and the methods are similar. For those interested, however, descriptions of methods are to be found in Acheson (1967, 1968).

Moreover, an epidemiologist or other worker collecting data that might be required for record linkage purposes should make himself aware of the method of identification of individuals in the particular files that he intends to use so that there is no difficulty in feeding his information into the file as required (see also Heasman, 1968).

Described here are the applications of record linkage in the field of epidemiology and the allied subjects of demography, social administration, genetics, etc. Brief consideration is given to the value of record linkage to the individual patient.

Before considering these applications, however, it should be stressed that the value of any particular set of linked data will depend upon the type of records that are held on file, the length of time the file has been in existence and the geographical area or population group whose records are held. Each of these factors is worth considering in some detail.

THE TYPE OF RECORDS

Most record linkage files in existence today have a basis either in hospital admission or in vital events (birth, marriage, death, etc.). It is generally agreed that the file which is likely to be of greatest use to the largest number of workers is that on which details of hospital in-patient treatment and death are held; it is upon this basis, indeed, that most of the examples of uses of record linkage mentioned in this chapter are given. For such a file to be of value, then, a very large proportion of all hospital admissions in the area must be covered, or at least the categories of exclusions must be well recognized and understood.

Registration of vital events is virtually complete in most developed countries today, so that the basis of a very useful medical record linkage file is available in those countries where, in addition, statistics based upon the collection of data from all hospital discharges are also produced.

Extension beyond vital events and hospital in-patient data depends very much upon the form of collection of other material and the resources available. Many of the possible extensions are difficult because of the sheer size of the problem. For example, out-patient and general practitioner consultations may outnumber in-patient admissions by a factor of ten and forty or more respectively, and this may well overload the organization. For such quantities of data to be held on a linked file is likely to strain even the largest resources, unless the particular file is of value locally for other purposes, particularly in the care of the individual patient (see below).

The inclusion of birth registration data in a linked file means that, with the exception of immigrants, the file should have an entry for each person in the population. Yet without some means of keeping individuals' addresses or areas of residence up-to-date the value of such a file as a population register is rather low. In some countries, however, notably in Scandinavia, individuals are required by law to notify changes of address, and by this means a complete and virtually up-to-date population register is available. The potentialities that this offers for the foundation of a record linkage file of value both to the individual patient and to the research worker are immense. Nevertheless, it should be remembered that there might well be insuperable barriers of confidentiality to its use in this respect. These same barriers will often preclude the use of population census data for record linkage purposes.

There is also something to say for the inclusion in the linked file of non-medical and non-demographic data. This might include, for example, contacts that individuals have with social welfare services. However, this again raises the problem of confidentiality. Once the purely medical and demographic fields are left behind there may be a not unreasonable fear in the minds of the public as to where the whole process is going to stop. Even within the medical field the utmost care must be taken to ensure that the principles of medical confidentiality are not breached. The traditions of the medical profession in this respect are strong and with adequate safeguards breaches are highly unlikely. For extension beyond the profession raises problems of interprofessional ethics which would need very close study and discussion before such a move should be permitted.

It therefore seems likely that a linked medical file covering a large geographical area will be limited in the number of different events that are recorded on it. With a smaller area more detailed coverage is possible, and when considering the establishment of a record linkage file the advantages of intensive coverage of a small area must be weighed against less detailed cover of a large one.

Other things being equal, there is no doubt that the wider the coverage the more value the linked file will have. This is so for two reasons: the mobility of the present-day population means that without wide geographical coverage individuals may very likely move beyond the limits of the area covered; and secondly, with wide coverage the likelihood is increased that the system of linked records may be incorporated into the previously existing medical information systems rather than be superimposed on them. Furthermore, the wider the coverage the more likely it is to coincide with other administrative boundaries.

It is conceivable for the future that local, regional, and national record linkage files will coexist with records of increasing summarization as centralization itself increases. The value of such multi-tiered files will need to be carefully assessed, however, if only because the problems of access and of confidentiality may make their use uneconomic.

The value of a record linkage file also increases with the length of time the file has been in existence. This is partly because the occurrence of related events in the same individual may be widely separated in time, for example the treatment of ankylosing spondylitis by radiotherapy and the subsequent development of leukaemia (Court-Brown and Doll, 1965). Moreover, the longer the time interval between one event and another the more difficult it is to trace an individual person, and the more chance there is that a linked file will provide the initial means of access to a patient's subsequent medical history.

USES IN MEDICAL CARE AND EPIDEMIOLOGY

Several possible classifications exist of the uses of record linkage but in this short review it is proposed to subdivide them into:

1. Statistical uses.
2. Uses for tracing individual records.
3. Their use for the treatment of individual patients.

STATISTICAL USES

Measurement of Morbidity

Under this heading are included those applications of record linkage which do not depend upon the identification of an individual 'outside' the computer and where the output is in numerical terms. Of course, for person-based statistics to be produced at all accurate linkage of individual event records has to be made.

Separate spells of hospital admission, attendances at an out-patient department or at a general practitioner's consulting room, however faithfully recorded, provide but a poor guide to the measurement of morbidity in the community, because the availability of services, the treatment policy and the needs of the patient all help to determine whether he has one or several contacts with the medical services for the same condition. Thus the number of hospital discharges (including deaths) for cancer of the lung is considerably greater than the number of deaths from the disease: in 1967 in Scotland discharges numbered 5,664 and deaths 3,150. The survival rate is known to be so low that the only reasonable explanation for the discrepancy in the figures is the repeated admission of the same individuals. Indeed, a check of 500 discharges of patients admitted to Scottish Hospitals in 1967 with a diagnosis of carcinoma of the bronchus revealed that only 341 individuals were involved. (These particular records were grouped by date of birth and related to patients aged between 34 and 42.)

With a linked file of medical data it becomes possible to discover how many individual patients have been involved, and thus to obtain a measure of incidence, provided that either all or at least a known proportion of people with the condition under scrutiny have records that are included in the linked file. Although it has been suggested that very few conditions are likely both to result in admission to hospital whenever they occur and also to be dealt with in one admission, there are a large number of conditions that almost inevitably result in hospital admission at some time during their course in a country with a high level of hospital provision (Heasman, 1965). Thus a linked system of hospital in-patient records covering a known geographical area should provide a measure of the incidence of a considerable proportion of the more serious end of the disease spectrum.

It should be noted, however, that this measurement of incidence is not immediately available on the establishment of the linked file, nor does the measure obtained comply strictly with the normally accepted sense of the term. To deal with the latter point first. If the file under scrutiny is one of linked hospital admissions then the measure of incidence will be related to that of the first admission of individuals with the condition being examined. Under normal circumstances, with no rapid change in treatment policy or in the true incidence of the disease, this will approximate closely to its actual incidence, for it seems a reasonable assumption that the variability in the stage of the disease at which hospital admission is found to be necessary will remain approximately constant. On the setting up of a linked file, however, the first admission of an individual after its establishment may not be the first admission with that disease, so that the first data available on persons under treatment will contain both new admissions and those over a previous period. After this initial period the number of first entries to the linked file will come closer and closer to the number of first admissions with the condition. The speed with which this figure approaches the true incidence will depend upon the mean duration of the disease prior to the event recorded, and upon its variance and the number of admissions of each person.

Two examples will help to clarify this. Acute appendicitis normally requires only one admission to hospital soon after the onset of the disease. Thus the true incidence of the disease will be calculable soon after the establishment of the linked file. With ulcerative colitis, on the other hand, with its relatively slow and highly variable onset and its large number of repeated admissions, some considerable period of time might elapse before data became available on the true incidence of the disease.

G

Studies of Prognosis

Linked data are often used for the statistical study of prognoses. A typical example of this is found in the survival rate studies carried out by many cancer registration schemes, for example the Registrar General (1958), where the patient's survival is noted at regular intervals following the initial registration until he either dies or is lost trace of. The most usual index of survival that is calculated from such data is the 5-year survival rate corrected to allow for mortality from causes other than the condition under review. The method is described by the Registrar General (1955). An approximate measure of prognosis is thus obtained, and analyses can be made according to different personal demographic or medical factors. With a general linked file this can be extended to many diseases very easily indeed. It should be noted, however, that although studies of this sort may provide a rough guide to the efficacy of different methods of treatment, they are not, and never can be, a substitute for properly controlled clinical trials. This is a point which is worth making, for in most statistical studies based upon data held in linked files, the occurrence of the initial event resulting in the entry of the record on the file and the subsequent history are dependent upon so many extraneous factors that only in rare instances will one be able to look to linked files for precise statistical data. Their value lies in the ease with which approximate measures of prognosis or incidence can be obtained, which without the existence of such a file might either be impossible or very difficult.

Apart from studies of survival, linked files containing the appropriate records can be used to obtain measures of hospital readmission rates, reoperation rates, etc., provided that these events occur within the geographical area covered by the linkage survey. Similarly the frequency with which two diseases occur in the same person at different periods of time can also be obtained. This emphasizes the argument for having as large an area as possible, for the readmission to the same hospital is usually easy to discover particularly with the unit record system that is now in general use. It is readmission to another hospital which is known only rarely. Studies involving admission to more than one hospital are of value in the administrative field (Hobbs and Acheson, 1966) and in providing a measure of total hospitalization.

In some countries the statistical records of mentally ill and obstetric patients are kept in different systems from that of the general hospital patient. However, the existence of a single file in which all types of hospital admission are held enables studies of the interrelationship of physical and mental disease to be carried out comparatively easily.

Thus far, the statistical uses considered have related to the linkage of records of different events in the same person, usually occurring at different periods of time[2] and possibly in different places.

Familial and Genetic Studies

Record linkage methods can also help considerably in bringing together the records of medical events occurring in the life of close relatives. For such linkage to be achieved, a link must be created 'across' the birth of an individual and must be held on the file. Normally this will be found in the birth certificate which should, for this purpose, contain sufficient identification data for both parents and child. Perhaps the most readily appreciated use in this context is the relationship of the antenatal period in the mother to that of the early life of her child. With hospital confinement becoming increasingly common and with good antenatal records kept, there should be little technical difficulty in relating these events with that of postnatal events in the child. Such data, particularly if available on a national scale, enable a very much broader survey of the relationship of disease and social factors in mother and child than is possible at the present time without considerable effort. Where systems of notification of congenital malformation are in existence the data may be linked to maternal records very easily.

Over longer periods of time the occurrence of diseases in both parents and offspring can be studied by means of family linkage files. One of the first projects studied by means of record linkage was that on patterns of fertility and family spacing (Newcombe and Rhynas, 1962).

The uses of computerized record linkage files for studies of disease and other events occurring over more than two generations must await the passage of time, but there is every reason to hope that linkage methods will considerably ease the study of human genetics and fertility.

USES FOR TRACING INDIVIDUAL RECORDS

Many of the statistical uses of record linkage will be of value in the provision of readily available, if approximate, measures. With increasing familiarity with longitudinal measures of morbidity (as opposed to single-event statistics) there is little doubt that their use will increase.

It is the author's opinion, however, that the most readily appreciated use of record linkage files will be the ease with which particular patients can be followed up. Naturally, the types of follow-up that are possible will depend on the records that are held on the file; it is almost essential that a record of death should be one of the items held.

The tracing of individual records can be done both prospectively and

[2] Different records of the same event may be of considerable interest, e.g. hospital records of death and the certificate of cause of death may contain differing and sometimes conflicting details (Alderson and Meade, 1967).

retrospectively. Prospective studies can be carried out by providing the organization responsible for the file with lists of individuals whom it is wished to follow up. These might include, for example, persons taking part in a long-term prospective clinical trial or who are suspected of having been exposed to industrial hazard; those who are to be followed up for observation of occurrence or recurrence of the disease under investigation.

This will be of value only if the occurrence of the disease is likely to be recorded on the file. For example, a study of a drug supposed to inhibit the onset of coronary thrombosis would be considerably facilitated by a linked file containing hospital admission and death records for this condition. On the other hand, such a file would be of little or no value in a study of the effect of an anti-influenzal vaccine.

It has been estimated that in Great Britain alone some 300,000 individuals are being followed up in order to investigate the occurrence or non-occurrence of particular forms of cancer. Such a follow-up would be rendered easy if the individuals were included on a linked file. In some instances, a simple note of occurrence of the particular event under study will be enough for the investigator, but in the majority of cases it is likely that he will require more detail than that held on the linkage file. On these occasions, when access is required either to the clinical record or to the patient, then the investigator need only be given the name of the hospital and/or of the physician in charge of the patient and the patient's case reference number. The investigator will then approach the particular hospital and request access to the case notes. In this way, responsibility for disclosure of medical details rests upon the patient's physician, and any breach of confidentiality is prevented. Should access to the patient or his relatives be required it should be granted only after the patient has given his permission to his physician. Even if the record file holds details of the patient's address it should not be given to the investigator unless the patient has previously given consent to such disclosure.

The entry of an individual's name on a record file will have to be made with as much of the identifying data (for example, social security number, date and place of birth) as the record linkage organization uses to effect matches. At regular intervals the list of individuals will be run against the other records held on the file and copies made of relevant details of hospital admissions or deaths. Provided that the geographical area is large enough and the admission to hospital is accurately recorded on the file, this use will save investigators much unrewarding labour in attempting to follow up patients whose subsequent medical history is of interest to them.

The retrospective use of record linkage files is essentially similar. In this case, the file will again be searched to produce summary records of the past history of patients in which the investigator is interested. It should be noted that this can be done either according to the name or other identification of the patient, or from lists of patients with a particular disease or in a particular occupation which can be easily obtained.

If the record linkage file has potential value to the investigator wishing to undertake a follow-up for epidemiological purposes, its value is at least as great for the clinical research worker who follows up his own cases. The methods used are identical. This application of record linkage is easily recognized and likely to be increasingly used; it also has value as a routine service in providing clinicians with summary details of the subsequent history of patients treated by them. Hubbard and Acheson (1967) have demonstrated that in only 37·9 per cent of cases was the death of a patient within 2 years of leaving hospital recorded in the clinical notes. Too often the subsequent history of a patient is unknown to his doctor. However, the routine provisions of details of deaths of patients dying outside the hospital of original treatment might bring about revision of treatment methods, if doctors were more aware of the long-term results of the treatment. Of considerable value in this connection would be the provision of data on return to work, by including social security and health insurance data on a file of linked records.

An administrative use of linked files of personal medical records has been demonstrated by Galloway (1966), in cases where an entry is made to the file on the birth of an individual. This record is then used at the appropriate time to form the basis of letters to parents requesting the infant's attendance for vaccination and immunization. As this is carried out the file is updated, or further effort can be made to contact those children not protected. An important effect of this procedure has been the unusually high immunization rate achieved (96 per cent for diphtheria, tetanus, and whooping cough). The file also forms the basis of up-to-date vaccination statistics and of providing payment for the doctors concerned. Similar methods are now being developed for inviting women to attend for cervical smear examinations, and there is no reason why such a file should not be used for other examinations, particularly those of vulnerable groups of the population, provided that the appropriate data are available with the addresses correctly recorded.

Finally, record linkage is further applied to the clearance of files with records relating to dead persons. With space increasingly at a premium in medical records departments, one way of relieving this problem is to remove records no longer needed. This can be achieved by notifying the hospital of the death of a person who was previously a patient there. Similar procedures will be of assistance to welfare and social security agencies.

THE VALUE OF RECORD LINKAGE TO THE INDIVIDUAL

Throughout this chapter, the emphasis has been placed upon the value of record linkage to the research worker, the clinician and his administrative colleagues. Does it have any potential of direct value to the individual patient?

At present, the answer seems to be that such value as it might have will necessarily be very limited, except as a means of facilitating surveillance (see above). This is because the sort of national or regional file that has been under consideration here will only contain very brief summary information on the individual. It will hold nothing like a complete medical record. Another important limitation is the difficulty of obtaining sufficient random access storage so that an individual's record will be available quickly enough for it to be of value to the clinician, for example, who wants to have it in hand within a period of time that he is prepared, or able, to wait for it. In this context five minutes may be too long for occasional use and five seconds too long for routine use. One long-term possibility, mentioned earlier, is that in the future there will be a national medical computer network. For this to be of any value, access to a record will have to be very rapid, which may offer insuperable technological problems. It seems likely, however, that even if problems of access can be overcome the restrictions placed upon the transmission of medical information by the need to maintain confidentiality makes such a system an unlikely eventuality.

It is conceivable that an unconscious patient, for example, whose name was known but whose medical history was not, might benefit from the ready accessibility of summary medical data held centrally. However, the number of occasions on which this would be of real value must be very small indeed, and in cost-benefit terms it would therefore be uneconomic.

Yet it should not be forgotten that, in the local hospital provided with a computer for the storage and processing of medical records, record linkage techniques must be used to ensure that the various reports, etc., which go to make up the medical record are brought together in one place in the computer record. However, there is a difference here from record linkage for a large region or country. In the local situation it must be ensured that linkage is carried out with a higher degree of certainty than need be the case when the primary object is research. When an individual patient depends upon a record linkage scheme for showing up such factors as drug sensitivity a wrong linkage could be a tragic affair.

The difference between record linkage on a national and regional basis and on a local (possibly hospital or health centre) basis is probably no more than one of degree, involving a difference of approach rather than of fundamental principle. Nevertheless it is a difference that should be borne in mind in any discussion of record linkage.

CONCLUSION

The organization of record linkage files is not expensive when considered alongside the cost of collecting the original data. Current experience of the (as yet incomplete) development in Scotland gives every reason to hope that the system's total development will be achieved for less than half the amount involved in the collection and processing of a single year's data. The problems may be greatly different in other situations, but the purpose of mentioning Scottish experience in this context is to stress that record linkage plans should not be ruled out because of cost factors without detailed study.

At the same time it should be stressed that the development of these files is still an act of faith. The full realization of their value cannot be appreciated for a considerable length of time, and then only if they are used by many workers in different situations. Time must therefore be allowed for the full development of record linkage and for as much experience in use as possible.

REFERENCES

ACHESON, E. D. (1967) *Medical Record Linkage*, London.

ACHESON, E. D., ed. (1968) *Record Linkage in Medicine*, Proceedings of the International Symposium, Edinburgh.

ALDERSON, M. R., and MEADE, T. W. (1967) Accuracy of diagnosis on death certificates compared with that in hospital records, *Brit. J. prev. soc. Med.*, 21, 22.

COURT-BROWN, W. M., and DOLL, R. (1965) Mortality from cancer and other causes after radiotherapy for ankylosing spondylitis, *Brit. med. J.*, 2, 1327.

DOLL, R., and HILL, A. B. (1964) Mortality in relation to smoking: ten years' observations of British doctors, *Brit. med. J.*, 1, 1399.

GALLOWAY, T. McL. (1966) Computers. Their use in local health administration, *Roy. Soc. Hlth J.*, 86, 213.

HEASMAN, M. A. (1965) Paper B. 3/I/E/28 prepared for World Population Conference, Belgrade, 1965.

HEASMAN, M. A. (1968) The use of record linkage in long-term prospective studies, in *Record Linkage in Medicine*, ed. Acheson, E. D., p. 251.

HOBBS, M. S. T., and ACHESON, E. D. (1966) Perinatal mortality and the organisation of obstetric services in the Oxford area in 1962, *Brit. med. J.*, 1, 499.

HUBBARD, M. R., and ACHESON, E. D. (1967) Notification of death occurring after discharge from hospital (Oxford Record Linkage Study), *Brit. med. J.*, 3, 612.

NEWCOMBE, H. B., and RHYNAS, P. O. W. (1962) *Proceedings of the Seminar on the Use of Vital and Health Statistics for Genetic and Radiation Studies*, United Nations, New York.

NEWCOMBE, H. B. (1965) Record linkage: concepts and potentialities, in *Mathematics and Computer Science in Biology and Medicine*, Medical Research Council, London, H.M.S.O., p. 43.

REGISTRAR GENERAL FOR ENGLAND AND WALES (1955) *Statistical Review for 1950–51*, London, H.M.S.O., p. 63.

REGISTRAR GENERAL FOR ENGLAND AND WALES (1958) *Statistical Review for 1953, Supplement on Cancer*, London, H.M.S.O.

STEWART, A., WEBB, J., and HEWITT, D. (1958) A survey of childhood malignancies, *Brit. med. J.*, 1, 1495.

8

FRENCH IDENTIFYING AND LINKING SYSTEMS

Louis M. F. Massé

IDENTIFICATION OF INDIVIDUALS FOR VARIOUS ADMINISTRATIVE PURPOSES AND RECORD LINKAGE IN SEVERAL FRENCH-SPEAKING AFRICAN COMMUNITIES

ONE of the principal problems facing social and medical research workers in developing countries is the correct identification of individuals for follow-up studies. The first section of this chapter describes the identification methods used in studies undertaken in the last two decades among some French-speaking African communities south of the Sahara. Very similar circumstances are found in other developing countries, and it is therefore hoped that interest in this discussion will not be limited to specialists in this particular geographical area.

Provided a long follow-up period is possible and the number of sampling units is limited, the problem of identification and retrieval can be solved very satisfactorily; results have sometimes been more encouraging than those obtained in highly developed countries. Such studies are not discussed here, but have been fully reported by Massé and Senecal (1961a and b), Massé (1962), Massé and Hunt (1963), and Massé (1969).

The following section is confined to a review of the work undertaken by different investigators in eight communities. It will be seen that in each case it has been necessary to adopt an empirical approach, evolving different identification methods to meet the particular local circumstances. An attempt is made to relate the methods used to the conditions in the area, to evaluate the results of the studies, and to draw some general conclusions about identification and record linkage.

NTEM, CAMEROUN (1949)

The Ntem area is situated in the southern part of the Cameroun, along the frontiers with Spanish Guinea, Gabon, and Congo. Its area is 35,000 square miles, and its population (1948) 147,000. Several censuses had been taken before 1949, but essentially for tax collection purposes; no attempt was made to relate these to other administrative files.

In 1949, Christol, Soupault, and Jourdan (Christol, 1951) began to set up a linkage system using three documents on an individual basis:

1. Identity card (with finger-prints).
2. Anthropometric files (with finger-prints).
3. Population files.

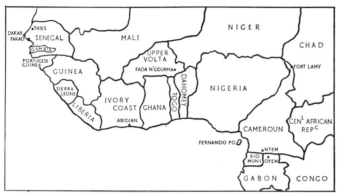

FIG. 1. Map of West Africa south of the Sahara, showing communities selected for study.

Linkage was obtained by two different numbers derived from the finger-print formula and the code number of the place of birth. Individual files were created by a team moving from village to village, carrying a mobile office which contained five different desks designed for:

1. Checking and handing out a set of three uncompleted cards to each individual.
2. Numbering the cards.
3. Completing the cards.
4. Finger-printing on identity and anthropometric card.
5. Rechecking and dispatching the three cards, one of which was given to the individual, another classified in the anthropometric files and the third in the population files.

It should be remembered that the setting up of files on an individual basis, without grouping by families, is rarely attempted; in this case it was decided to note the parents' numbers on the children's cards. Updating of these files did not appear too difficult a task. Several linkages were derived from these central files at various levels (village, canton, subdivision, and region), with the administrative services (census, justice, civil status registration, and voting list).

This work has now unfortunately been discontinued. It is obvious that the devices used for identification of individuals, and associated files, were too complex and time-consuming. It is, however, important to bear in mind that this attempt was made twenty years ago. Later on, many methods, sometimes refined, were employed in the same area to obtain vital statistics using sampling processes, but no very reliable results were obtained.

THIÈS, SENEGAL (1953)

A population census of the city of Thiès (Senegal, ex-French West Africa) was undertaken in April 1953, when 50,000 inhabitants were recorded. A sociodemographic investigation on a random sampling basis was then carried out by Massé and Mercier (Massé, 1954, 1956 and 1957).

The sampling units chosen were heads of families and fell into three categories, 'married male heads of families', 'female heads of families', and 'singles'. The main problem faced in the investigation was the retrieval for interviewing of individuals drawn in the sample. At that time the houses in the city of Thiès were not numbered, and most of the streets had neither name nor number. It was therefore impossible in most cases to identify an individual by his address. In addition, many names and surnames in the area are similar, and, when written in Latin letters, their spelling is uncertain. Gambia (then a British Protectorate) is not far from Thiès, and the alternative French–Latin or English–Latin spellings of some usual Sengalese Moslem surnames like Mamadou, Amadou, Hamaduh, Ahmed, and Mohamed, is an interesting topic for discussion among armchair epidemiologists indulging in combinatory analysis, but is of very little help in the field.

After various unsuccessful attempts to find a suitable method of identification, it was decided to write a complete list for every sampling unit of the names of the household inhabitants, with parental relationships, sex and age (approximate) as registered in the census. The list included the wife or wives, the children of each wife, other relatives and any other inhabitants of the household. The list was in itself the identifying device. Part of this list was given to the interviewer to enable him to find the interviewee, and, when he returned to the central mobile office, a comparison between the remaining part of the list and the family structure recorded in the forms of the sociodemographic investigation allowed the supervisor to check that the proper sampling unit had been contacted. The more complex the household, the easier the identification of the head of a family became. For example, a polygamous married man with two or three wives living in the same household was easier to identify than a monogamous one, since it was considered very unlikely that two synonymous men of similar age would marry two synonymous women of similar age. For the same reason, identification became progressively easier as the number of children belonging to each wife increased.

The identification methods used in Thiès were, in fact, unexpectedly successful for the first sample of 700 heads of families. It was, however, slow, tedious, and expensive; but after several similar investigations in other cities it was possible to refine the identification method. After a while some of the interviewers began to use the official informant of the survey in a more effective way, and to use a set of parallel informants through the local channels of microsocial gossip. Those interviewers who obtained better results by doing this were kept in the team for other surveys. They began to develop their own methods, being quickly able to select the right informant. Consequently it was possible, at least where the Wolof language was used, to discover nearly every individual in the community, even with poor identifying data.

DAKAR, SENEGAL (1960)

The identification method described above was used by Massé and Pène to recover individuals admitted during the previous five years to Le Dantec Hospital (Dakar) for infectious hepatitis. Dakar had at that time 300,000 inhabitants.

The results of the retrieval process were very satisfactory, even though the initial identifying data found in the files of the hospital were limited to the following items:

1. Name and surname.
2. Sex.
3. Age (approximate).
4. Marital status (subject to change).
5. Address (approximate and subject to change).
6. Date of admission and discharge from hospital.

The retrieval of individuals through this sociocultural device of identification in fact proved to be one of the most interesting features of the study.

FAKAO, SENEGAL (1956 AND 1965)

The sociodemographic uses of Catholic parish records (baptism, marriage, and burial) have been recognized for some time. In some areas of the world, such records have been in existence for centuries: in Sienna they can be traced back to 1379, and in Nantes to 1416.

In 1953, an unpublished government report stressed the advantages of using such records (Massé, 1953). The conclusions reached in the report were based on data obtained from Southern Senegal, and may be summarized as follows:

In areas where the Catholic missions are established the local administrators could make good use of the data abstracted from the parish records
in their annual reports. They would then have several important advantages,
for the following reasons:

1. Parish records are on the whole well kept by missionaries.
2. Missionaries have a good knowledge of the ages of the local inhabitants
   (from christening dates, except in the case of converts) and are also
   well informed about the origins of the inhabitants and the nature of
   the union from which the children originate.
3. A reliable register of the mission population is available.
4. Some of the missions cover a very well-bounded territory, defined by
   natural boundaries such as streams or forests.
5. Each birth is recorded at the time of baptism; eventual death is also
   recorded on the birth record.
6. Each death is noted on the burial record.

The final point emphasized by the report was that this source of information
should not be underestimated by government statisticians, some of whom
maintained that the only valid information was that obtained by random
sampling surveys under their exclusive supervision. These statisticians were
later forced to admit that their survey procedure was, in fact, generally
inefficient in many of the situations found in developing countries.

However, despite the advantages of the parish record system quoted above,
the results obtained from these sources were still unsatisfactory after ten
years' research (Massé, 1966). The probable explanation was that the correct
methods of improving one source of data by linkage with another were not
available at that time.

The project was therefore abandoned, but was recently readopted using a
record linkage system. The latest study (Lacombe, 1968) was carried out in
a small island, Fakao, which was selected for the remarkably good book-
keeping of its parish records. The island constitutes part of a remote scattered
village, Palmarin, and is situated on the Atlantic coast, 100 miles south of
Dakar.

The principal types of data linked in this study were parish records, civil
status registration and census data, and a retrospective investigation of births
and deaths was also carried out. The parish records were of four kinds—
christening, marriage, burial, and confirmation—and covered 5,000 past
events. The census was taken in January 1966 and involved the whole population of the island. The retrospective investigation was carried out after the
linkage of census and parish records, and aimed to trace the people mentioned
in the parish records who did not appear on the census forms, to investigate
the obstetric history of the women, and to make a comparison with existing
data on the census and parish records. The main interest of this linkage system

lies in the fact that it was based almost exclusively on family ties derived from births and marriages, and 'even the Christian names could not be used with any certainty for linkage, since many people would forget them and use the local names' (Lacombe, 1968).

This type of work, which uses extremely limited identifying data, is thought possible only in very small communities, and Lacombe himself admits that it would be very difficult to adopt it for use among larger, developing populations. If, however, an attempt were made to expand this method to cover a larger community, using a computer, it would certainly be found ultimately that the identifying device was an index number based only on sex, date of birth, and dates of birth and marriage of parents.

It is interesting to note the last point that Lacombe emphasizes:

'It is the first time that a study of parish records in French-speaking Africa yields reliable results on mortality, infant mortality, perinatal mortality, fertility, offspring size, etc. The reason for this success is the linkage process.'

FADA N'GOURMA, UPPER VOLTA (1965)

In this area Baudin carried out an experiment in the identification of leprous patients. At first a serial number was used, but as this alone did not prove to be entirely satisfactory, the *Service des Grandes Endémies* decided to use some other information in order to make a more precise identification of every individual concerned. This method again failed to be entirely reliable. The names of the parents were then added, and two files were created, one by serial number and another by village. This breakdown by village had both an operational usefulness and an identifying power, for it decreased the number of synonyms in every section of the file.

OYEM, GABON (1967)

In this district, which was an entirely new one, Baudin carried out a further study using the same type of files as in Fada n'Gourma. Some modifications in the system were made to improve the identifying power of the files. The size of the files was considerably reduced and all unnecessary documents eliminated. They were also classified according to disease pattern and the route followed by the three different teams working on screening, treatment, and follow-up. Subfiles were kept for special cases, for example, death and error of diagnosis, and for those withdrawn, unknown, or cured.

CHAGOUA, CHAD (1967)

The different investigations described above all illustrate the difficulty of finding reliable identifying data for individuals in developing communities.

It is therefore tempting to use other devices to facilitate the retrieval of individual files. In a W.H.O. study now in progress in Chagoua, a suburb of the city of Fort Lamy, medals are being used; a single medal displaying a unique identifying number is given to each individual in the community (Vernier and Seguin, personal communication).

There are several difficulties involved in the use of this device. The first is one of acceptability. In this particular area acceptability is good, and as a result the people soon discovered the advantage the device brought to a proper use of the health services. The second problem is to find a material strong enough to be carried daily without being lost or damaged. The third problem is one of duration, and relates to the type of numbering system used. If, for example, this is partly derived from the number of the house, the appropriate number becomes obsolete every time the family moves. If the system is partly derived from the family number, based on, for example, marriage, it becomes obsolete whenever a young person begins to live independently of his family. Finally, if the system is partly derived from the age group of the individual, it will inevitably become obsolete in a few years.

The only valid system is to adopt an index number derived from the permanent characteristics of the individual concerned: that is, sex, date of birth (if the individual receives the number while quite young or a civil registration system exists), place of birth, and ethnic group. These last two items necessitate the construction of a special code for the area.

ABIDJAN, IVORY COAST (1968)

The use of finger-prints for identification, first introduced on a pilot scale in Cameroun by Christol (1951), has recently been renewed by Italian investigators with the help of more advanced electronic material. Furthermore, in order to detect pluralism of salaries in government agencies, a method of identification by finger-print has been proposed for civil servants, to link individuals on different payrolls. Hitherto, this system has been judged more expensive than budget wastage, and has therefore not been used for record linkage.

CONCLUSION

In all the studies described above different identification methods were used. The European and North American practice of using the surname as the principal identifying device has in some places been incorporated into the identification system, but it often proved impossible to use either first name or surname. In many places names are uncertain and it was therefore found necessary to increase the identifying power of names with other data.

In Thiès, household listing was used (Massé, 1954, 1956 and 1957); in Oyem, the routes followed by the research workers were incorporated into the system. This last innovation is comparable to the methods used by electricity and water supply plants in highly developed urban areas, where the identifying number of each customer is derived from his surname and his position on the service itinerary.

However, the most efficient method of identification yet devised for developing countries is the finger-print system, which has been tentatively used in Ntem, Cameroun (Christol, 1951) and Abidjan, Ivory Coast. Finger-prints are, in many ways, the direct counterpart of the signature, being unique for every individual, and a finger-print system of identification therefore renders unnecessary any supplementary information dependent on literacy or a reliable knowledge of personal data. But until the next generation of computers has been developed, when it will be possible to process such data automatically at a reasonably low cost, the general introduction of any identification system depending on finger-print material will present insuperable problems.

Where reliable information on dates of birth and marriage is available, as in Fakao, a complex system can be evolved based on both familial (date of marriage) and individual (date of birth) numerical data. Lacombe's work in Fakao (1968) underlines the need for introducing a record linkage system in dealing with data derived from Catholic files, for whereas very satisfactory results have been produced in Fakao, many attempts in other areas to use similar resources without the use of a record linkage system have proved unsuccessful.

IDENTIFICATION AND RECORD LINKAGE IN FRENCH-SPEAKING EUROPEAN COMMUNITIES

In the absence of published data for the French-speaking areas of Switzerland or Belgium, this section will be principally concerned with the present situation in France. Although a plan for the development of a record linkage system in Belgium was begun in 1965, results are not yet available.

In France, most record linkage studies are dependent on the national index number which has now been in use for nearly thirty years. In 1940 the *Service de la Démographie* was created. In 1941 *Repertoires* were established at the eighteen regional centres, and were intended to identify every individual born after 1881. The index number used included sex (one digit), city of birth (two digits), month of birth (two digits), department of birth (two digits), and a three-digit serial number. It is surprising that these identification repertoires were not used by the French and German police between 1941 and 1944; during that period the information obtained was, in fact, used only for linking the various records relating to civil status registration. This was particularly necessary at a time when the mobility of the population was considerably increased by the effect of the war.

The epidemiological uses of the national index number have been discussed by Massé (1970).

THE USE OF THE NATIONAL INDEX NUMBER IN A STUDY OF MORTALITY BY OCCUPATION

In a study of differences in mortality by occupation (Calot and Febvay, 1965; Calot, 1969) a sample of adult males was selected from the 1954 census. The following criteria were used in the selection:

1. Nationality (a French citizen, born in France).

2. Sex (males, and the wife of every married male selected).

3. Age. (As the main variable studied was occupation, it was important to avoid the selection of young people particularly liable to changes in occupation. The sample therefore included only those who were between 30 and 70 years of age in 1954.)

4. Occupation. (It was considered necessary to select the sample from a limited number of occupational groups, so that occupation should be:

    i. homogeneous within the group

    ii. unconnected to a specific age group and not subject to change with the age of the individual

    iii. unaffected by changes in definition in the last decades—for example, 'mechanic'.)

Twelve occupational groups were chosen and in theory 50,000 individuals could have been drawn from each of the groups; in practice about 41,000 were selected. Variable sampling fractions were used according to age and occupation (for example, 1/1 for teachers and Catholic priests and 1/195 for workers aged 65–69). The total sample was expected to reach 600,000; in fact it included 500,000 individuals.

Individuals drawn in the sample were identified at the *Repertoire National d'Identification* with the help of the national index number. Identification proved to be impossible for 16,576 persons (3·46 per cent of the total sample, with differences between the various occupational groups, misidentifications being rare for farmers, teachers, and priests, and high for clerks and unskilled labourers). In addition, the initial census form was illegible at least in part for 1·72 per cent of the sample.

There are two different standpoints from which the relationship between mortality and occupation may be considered:

1. In a study of 'professional mortality', when death occurs as a direct result of work hazards.

2. In a study of mortality within an 'occupational group', when there is no clear causal association between death and work conditions.

The assessment of 'professional mortality' presents relatively few problems, since death occurs during employment and there is therefore little doubt about the true occupation of the deceased or the cause of death. The measurement of mortality within an 'occupational group' is, however, a much more difficult task. In developed countries the individuals relevant to this type of study generally die some time after retirement, and the occupation notified on the death certificate is, therefore, often vague. The deceased may also have taken up some subsidiary employment after retirement age, and could then very easily be classified according to his last, short-term occupation. In this case the information recorded on the death certificate is definitely misleading.

In order to obtain valid results in any study of an occupational group it is essential to relate the circumstances of death (i.e. age, place, cause, etc.) on the death certificate to the occupation declared before retirement age. In the study by Calot and Febvay the obvious source for the second set of data was the national census of 1954, which was undertaken five years before the commencement of the investigation when all individuals eligible for the sample were 70 or younger and in permanent employment. Information from death certificates was therefore linked with the census data.

This study is the most comprehensive investigation of the relationship between mortality and occupation yet undertaken in France. The only other comparable studies have been limited to very restricted age groups (for example, Croze, 1963).

THE USE OF THE NATIONAL INDEX NUMBER IN AN ANALYSIS OF THE EFFICIENCY OF THE HEALTH SERVICES

The social security system in France is divided into several district *régimes* with independent financial status. Some of these regimes deal with a very restricted section of the population (for example, railway workers, miners, farmers, etc.), but the main regime—the *régime général*—deals with 30,000,000 beneficiaries. As the *régime général* is an insurance system covering 80 per cent of individual expenditure on hospitals, drugs, surgery, and general practitioner consultations, the amount of information handled by the organization is enormous, which has deterred several investigators from using this material for epidemiological research. In November 1965 a national investigation was begun, however, using the national index number as the identifying device and taking a sample drawn on a 1/12 to 1/120 basis (Sanson Carette, 1966). It is thought that this system of identification should be operating smoothly by 1970.

H

THE USE OF THE NATIONAL INDEX NUMBER IN
EPIDEMIOLOGICAL FOLLOW-UP STUDIES

In 1960 Professor Schwartz of the *Institut National de la Santé et de la Recherche Medicale* (I.N.S.E.R.M.) established a service for French doctors interested in obtaining follow-up information on their patients for research purposes. The cost to the individual is small, being only a shilling for an indication of whether the subject is still alive, a shilling for the 'last known address' and two shillings for 'continuous surveillance and notification of date and place of death'. The main users of this repertoire are cancer registries (which have required information on more than 70,000 individuals), research workers involved in prospective studies (information required for more than 25,000) and those interested in industrial hygiene, for example, workers exposed to nuclear radiation (information required for 13,000). This repertoire offers to epidemiologists the most efficient national system of linkage yet devised in France.

THE NATIONAL INDEX NUMBER AND MEDICAL RECORD
LINKAGE

The 'Guihard' files are records of admission to all private clinics and public hospitals in the city of Rennes. They were set up in 1958 by Dr. Guihard and are at present kept by a small clerical staff. It is, however, hoped that their possible uses will expand with the use of a computer rented by the School of Public Health. The files are classified according to individual patients, and hitherto the main identification system has been based on surname, christian name, and address. From now on the French national index number will be used, and it is hoped that within a few years all the 650,000 inhabitants of the *Ille et Vilaine* department will be included in this system.

CONCLUSION

The national index number has now been in existence in France for nearly thirty years, but it should be stressed that for the first two decades its use was almost exclusively confined to a small number of administrative tasks (i.e. linkage of civil status records, voting lists, etc.). During the last decade, the value of the index number for social and medical research purposes has been realized, though its use has so far been restricted to a very few studies. The most important of these have been discussed in this section. So far, the index number has not been used for work involving income tax, police investigations and records, and other legal aspects of civil administration.

The increasing availability of computers has revealed new areas of possible use, but two basic problems must be resolved before a comprehensive national system of record linkage can be introduced. The first is technical: the index number must be changed, and probably simplified. A national system of record linkage is now successfully in operation in the Scandinavian countries, and the results obtained there could provide a useful model for the proposed French system. The second problem is ethical and involves the question of confidentiality: the possible abuses of such a system and the threat to individual freedom.

RECORD LINKAGE IN FRENCH-SPEAKING COMMUNITIES OF AMERICA

There is as yet no evidence from the French-speaking countries of Central America of any contribution to the development of record linkage. By contrast, the French-speaking community of Canada in the Quebec province provides ideal conditions for experiments in record linkage. The quality of available data, the proportion of the population covered, and the length of the coverage period are probably unequalled in any other country of the world.

CIVIL STATUS REGISTRATION IN QUEBEC

Parish records for christenings, burials, and marriages have been kept by Catholic priests in Quebec for more than three hundred years. Although the same practice is adopted in many other Catholic countries, Quebec is one of the few areas where they have not been destroyed by repeated wars. It is therefore possible to trace the genealogies of the majority of the French Canadian population from the time of immigration. Except for the early period, there are two copies of all parish records, one remaining in the parish district and the other sent to the local judicial centre.

The value of these records for research purposes has been appreciated for some considerable time, and various attempts have been made to collate and analyse them. In 1870 Tanguay began to trace the genealogies of the French Canadian immigrant families, beginning with the first settlers and continuing until 1760. Langlois (1934) made a statistical analysis of Tanguay's data, and twenty years later Professor Henripin (1954) of Montreal University carried out a further analysis of the material for a study of historical demography.

Professor Laberge (Department of Genetics, Laval University, Quebec) has concentrated on the most recent years of registration and has undertaken several genetic studies in co-operation with the *Service de la Demographie du Ministère de la Santé*.

The *Institut Drouin*, a private firm specializing in genealogies, has a microfilm copy of all parish records for the whole three hundred years of registration. If public funds were made available for its use, this could be a very useful source of information for research.

Without this financial backing, Charbonneau and Legaré (1967a and b; 1969) found themselves unable to use the records of the *Institut* and undertook to build up a complete microfilm copy of all parish records up to 1850. The first section, covering the years before 1765, has now been completed and gives a record of some 27,000 events. These are filed on an individual basis, with an index number for record linkage purposes. The results of their study have been made available as a 'data bank' for other research workers.

The index number allows a cross-check to be made between civil status registration and successive censuses. Censuses were first taken in Quebec in 1666 and 1667 (probably the first modern censuses in the world), and the work of record linkage with civil registration starts with data recorded for 1 January 1667. This linkage process is time-consuming, but while it is in progress the collection of microfilmed parish records for the years 1765–1850 is continuing.

During the early period of settlement, some of the names recorded are uncertain, as the practice of changing one's name was then comparatively common. To a lesser extent this situation resembles that described in Fakao (Lacombe, 1968), and further cross-checks based on dates of birth and marriage have been devised to ensure correct identification.

HOSPITAL DATA IN THE QUEBEC PROVINCE

All patients admitted to hospital and to most private clinics are covered by a government insurance plan. This is, in fact, true of the whole of Canada. For all admissions a form is sent to the Ministry of Health for refund. These forms include details of admission, discharge, length of stay, diagnosis, prescriptions, surgery, name and ward of the physician in charge, and a breakdown of the cost of medical care. Other non-medical items, such as civil status and social class characteristics are also included. Data processing is carried out by a Ministry Unit and analyses are undertaken either by the Ministry or by affiliated scientists at the local universities. The information is generally analysed by hospital ward or physician, an analysis which is principally concerned with hospital management, zoning, and cost. Up to now there has been no attempt to link these admissions on an individual basis: every admission is considered separately, and two successive admissions of the same individual to the same or different hospitals are at present unrelated. Individually linked records are now, however, required by the Ministry for the analysis of the cost of care. Several types of index number have been proposed, and an individual linkage system could be in operation within a few years.

CONCLUSION

It seems highly probable that in the near future Montreal University will have evolved a complete record linkage system for all the vital events of the French Canadian population. These records will cover a period of three hundred years, and those for successive generations will be linked. At the same time, all medical records, which include diagnostic data, will be filed in the Ministry computer. Once these records have been linked on an individual basis it will be possible to relate the two sets of data. As the population of the Quebec province is relatively small, it is ideally suited to the present capacity of the computer, and linkage would present few problems.

This proposed linkage system would benefit epidemiological research projects in two ways. Firstly, in any study requiring information on both hospital admissions and vital statistics, it would be possible to process all the data simultaneously. Secondly, it would be possible to analyse the genealogy of patients suffering from genetic diseases (porphyria, for example) or from any disease in which a genetic factor is involved. The aim would then be to trace one or more common ancestors among the subjects studied. Once such common ancestors were found, all descendants could be identified, and an examination could be made of those still living in order to determine any unusual patterns of morbidity among this selected population. An entirely new type of epidemiological investigation would then become possible. Once this historical linkage process was evolved, the same type of study, using a modified system of analysis, could be undertaken for all conditions in which a familial factor is involved. There are few conditions for which a study of this kind would not be valuable.

In this type of study, the only limiting factors are likely to be the availability of financial resources and of scientists qualified to carry out the analyses of the collected data. The quality of material available for study and the facilities for data processing are unlikely to present problems.

In view of the population size of the Quebec province, the relative stability of the French Canadian population and the quality of local medical care and recording, this area provides unique opportunities for the epidemiologist, particularly for the study of familial or genetic conditions.

REFERENCES

CALOT, G., and FEBVAY, M. (1965) La mortalité différentielle selon le milieu social, *Etudes et Conjuncture*, No. 11, I.N.S.E.E., Paris.

CALOT, G. (1969) *L'Analyse de la Mortalité Différentielle. Présentation Méthodologique de Quelques Travaux Réalisés en France*, communication presentée au Congrès de l'Union Internationale pour l'Etude Scientifique de la Population, London.

CHARBONNEAU, H., and LEGARÉ, J. (1967a) La démographie historique au Canada, *Recherches Sociodémographiques, VIII (mai-août)*.

CHARBONNEAU, H., and LEGARÉ, J. (1967b) La population du Canada aux recensements de 1666 et 1667, *Population*, **22**, No. 6 (*nov.-dec.*).

CHARBONNEAU, H., and LEGARÉ, J. (1969) *La Démographie Historique au Canada Français avant 1800*, Congrès de l'Union Internationale pour l'Etude Scientifique de la Population, London.

CHRISTOL, J. (1951) Un essai de fichier démographique au Cameroun, *I.N.S.E.E. Serie Etudes*, Supplément No. 20.

CROZE, M. (1963) *La Mortalité Infantile selon le Milieu Social*, communication présentée au Congrès de l'Union Internationale pour l'Etude Scientifique de la Population, Ottawa.

HENRIPIN, J. (1954) *La Population Canadienne au débout du XVIIIième Siècle*, P.U.F., Paris.

LACOMBE, B. (1968) *Fakao (Sénégal) Depouillement de Registres Paroisieaux et Enquête Démographique Rétrospective*, O.R.S.T.O.M., Paris.

LANGLOIS, G. (1934) *Histoire de la Population Canadienne-française*, Montreal.

MASSÉ, G., and SENECAL, J. (1961a) Etude des différences de l'épaisseur du pli cutane chez les nourissons atteints ou exempts de signes de carence nutritionnelle, *Bull. Soc. med. Afr. noire Langue franç.*, **6**, 706.

MASSÉ, G., and SENECAL, J. (1961b) Variations saisonnières de quelques mensurations chez le nourisson dakerois, *Bull. Soc. med. Afr. noire Langue franç.*, **6**, 711.

MASSÉ, G. (1962) Comparaison de la maturation osseuse chez de jeunes enfants de Dakar et de Boston, in *Modern Problems in Pediatrics, Vol. VII, Croissance de l'Enfant Normal pendant les Trois Premières Années*, ed. Merminod, A., Basel, p. 199.

MASSÉ, G., and HUNT, E. E. (1963) Skeletal maturation of the hand and wrist in West African children, *Hum. Biol.*, **35**, 1.

MASSÉ, G. (1969) *Croissance et Developpement de l'Enfant à Dakar*, publication du Centre International de l'Enfance.

MASSÉ, L. (1953) Projet d'étude démographique des pays peu connus, *Memoire de l'Institut Français d'Afrique Noire*, Dakar.

MASSÉ, L. (1954) Enquêtes et sondages sociodémographiques en zones urbaines d'Afrique Occidentale Français, in *Comptes rendues du Congrès Mondial de la Population*, Vol. 5, Sc. 15 and 21, Rome, p. 175.

MASSÉ, L. (1956) Contribution a l'étude de la ville de Thiès. Note concernant un sondage sociodémographique. Premier dépouillement numérique sur la situation matrimoniale, *Bulletin de l'Institut Français d'Afrique Noire*, T.XVIII, Ser.B, Nos. 1 and 2 (*jan.-avr.*), p. 255.

MASSÉ, L. (1957) Contribution à l'étude de la ville de Thiès. (II) Suite du dépouillement numérique sur la situation matrimoniale (extrait d'un sondage sociodémographique), *Bulletin de l'Institut Français d'Afrique Noire*, T.XIX, Ser.B, Nos. 1 and 2 (*jan.-avr.*), p. 275.

MASSÉ, L. (1966) *Seasonal Differences in Health Status in some West African Urban Communities*, Dr. P. H. Dissertation, Harvard University School of Public Health, Cambridge, Mass.

MASSÉ, L. (1970) National index number as a tool for research in epidemiology, *Proceedings of the Fifth Scientific Meeting of the International Epidemiological Association, Primosten, Yugoslavia.*

SANSON CARRETTE, A. (1966) *Rapport sur les Statistiques Annuelles de Depenses et de Dénombrements de l'Assurance Maladie*, mimeographed report, Ministry of Social Affairs, Paris.

TANGUAY, C. (1870) *Dictionnaire Généalogique des Familles Canadiennes*, Montreal.

PART V

DATA PROCESSING

9

DATA PROCESSING FOR A PRIVATE CENSUS

A. E. Beñnett and H. S. Kasap

A UNIQUE opportunity for studies in the local community was provided by
the recent reorganization of hospital and specialist services in the area of St.
Thomas's Hospital. This general reorganization coincided with the rebuilding
of the hospital itself, and it was felt that the planning of both projects would
be advanced by studies on the prevalence and incidence of important chronic
diseases and a measurement of the use made of medical services.

Preliminary studies of patients attending the hospital (Bennett, 1966;
Montgomery, 1968) showed that the majority lived in the surrounding densely
populated area. The area chosen for the community studies was defined as
the six northern electoral wards in the Greater London Borough of Lambeth.
At the time of the last national census in 1961 this area held a population of
approximately 100,000 persons (General Register Office, 1963).

As there was no valid sampling frame for the identification of stratified
random samples of the population, the first step was to perform a sample
census. The main part of the programme comprised four major field surveys,
to be completed in under thirty months. With this schedule it was obvious
that close attention had to be paid to methods of data collection and handling.
It was a logical extension of previous work to minimize all clerical and other
manual procedures and to resort to automated methods of data processing
and storage using a computer. This chapter describes the methods designed for
the conduct of a large-scale private census.

SAMPLE

In 1966 a one-in-five random sample of dwellings in the defined area was
prepared by the Census Office of the General Register Office. This was drawn
from the list of dwellings and institutions constructed from the National
Census in 1961. In April 1966 a national one-in-ten sample census was performed; the sample for our survey was drawn in the same way, but not
overlapping the sample for the nation-wide operation.

In a national census individuals present at a specified date and time are
required by law to complete a return; by contrast, our survey was dependent
on co-operation obtained by invitation and had to take place over a period of

time. It was decided to eliminate hospitals and hotels from the sample, and also other institutions where it would be difficult to define the permanently resident population. As the primary objective was to create a sampling frame of residents in the area for the conduct of further studies, and not to conduct a total enumeration, these eliminations were considered allowable. A definition of 'normally resident' was introduced into the protocol to allow for the inclusion of individuals temporarily absent from their main place of residence during the time of the survey.

The next task undertaken was to identify and delete all property that had been demolished between 1961 and 1966. This involved considerable field work as each dwelling had to be viewed. To facilitate this and the field work of the census operation, the area was divided into five convenient working units, each unit being the responsibility of one member of the permanent field work staff. New dwellings erected since 1961 were identified and sampled from the valuation lists of the Borough Council.

The original sample of dwellings contained 5,640 addresses, from which 326 demolished properties were deleted, and to which 432 new sample addresses were added. The task for completion therefore was to collect and record data on residents in 5,746 dwellings.

For data processing each dwelling was allocated a numerical code. The first digit identified the electoral ward, the next three the street name and postal district code, and the last three the house or dwelling number. Large blocks of apartments with individual names and numbering systems were given a unique three-digit code in place of the street code, identifying the block together with the street and postal district code. An eighth digit allowed coding of similarly numbered addresses with separate dwellings identified individually by a letter, for example 9a, 9b, etc.; a ninth and tenth digit allowed for internally numbered dwellings within the same numbered address. The method of data collection and processing required that address codes were created and allocated before the start of the field work.

METHOD

It was desired to collect the full names, sex, and dates of birth of all persons involved; for adults, information was required on their occupation—for social class classification—marital status, age of school leaving, country of birth, hospital attendance in the previous six months, data on the presence of disability and impairment, and the name of the general practitioner with whom they were registered. To record these data, a large folded form was designed, modelled on that used for the national census, with space for the entry of data for six individuals. It was intended that data would be extracted on to coding sheets for the preparation of punch cards for computer input.

A full-scale pilot trial of this form achieved a totally unsatisfactory response rate of 79 per cent completed. In view of this, the methods of data recording and the field-work procedure were completely revised. Questions relating to country of birth and name of general practitioner were dropped and year of birth was substituted for full date of birth. This last modification subsequently proved to be a serious mistake, as full date of birth provides important data for identifying and linking together records belonging to the same person.

To record these data two forms were designed. The first of these was an enumeration form for recording the identifying data of sex, year of birth, and full name of each person; the second was a short self-administered questionnaire containing questions on marital status, occupation, school leaving age, hospital attendance as an in-patient, out-patient or casualty patient, and the presence of disability or impairment. This questionnaire was deliberately kept short and simple to achieve as high a co-operation rate as possible.

The plan of the field work required that two visits were made to each address at an interval of a week. Before the start of field work, a form for each address in the sample was prepared with actual address and coded address in the appropriate spaces. The forms then served as instructions to the field workers on which dwellings to enumerate. At the first visit the field worker completed the enumeration form shown in FIGURE 2. For each person resident at the address, a line was completed recording sex as M or F, year of birth omitting the first digit 1, forenames in full with each name separated by an asterisk, and surname. Each letter, digit, or asterisk was entered into a single box representing one column on a conventional eighty-column punch card. If the number of letters and spaces needed to record the forenames exceeded twenty, the first two names were recorded in full and the third and any other names were abbreviated to their initial letters. Married couples were identified by bracketing their names to enable wives to be classified according to social class from their husbands' occupations. The names of individuals to whom questionnaires were delivered were noted on the extreme right of the enumeration form by the entry of a tick in the appropriate column.

Every form had a unique four-digit number and each row was numbered, so that an entry along a line of a form was automatically allocated a unique five-digit code number. The form allowed for up to ten entries. When every person resident at the address had been entered, the field worker signed the form to indicate completeness. After checking for legibility and obvious errors it was then passed directly to the punch card operator for the preparation of one punch card per person.

At the same visit a questionnaire for recording the other personal data was left for completion by every person born in 1951 or before, that is, aged $15\frac{1}{2}$ years or older. Despite the disadvantages of recording only the year of birth, this practice at least ensured that the minimum age was precisely and easily identified by the field workers. The questionnaires were collected at a second

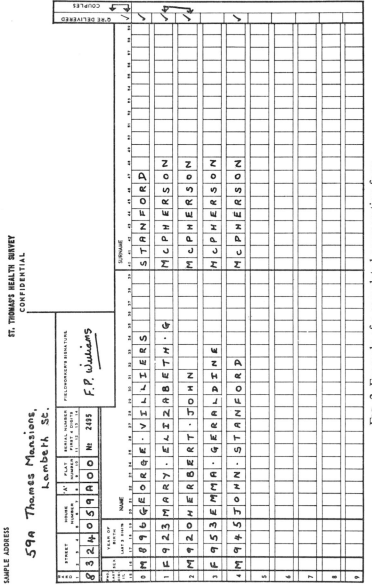

Fig. 2. Example of a completed enumeration form.

visit one week later. As the completed enumeration forms were immediately withdrawn from the field for data processing they were no longer available to identify where the second visits were to be made. A field-work card was therefore prepared from each enumeration form containing the names and addresses of individuals to whom questionnaires had been delivered.

The questionnaire, on completion, contained the address code, the person's unique number, year of birth and replies to the questions. These data were subsequently coded and transferred to a punch card. Thus, for every person identified in the census a punch card was prepared containing address, number, full name, sex, and year of birth. For every person over $15\frac{1}{2}$ years of age, a second punch card was prepared containing the questionnaire data. Each of these cards also contained the encoded address and the five-digit identifying number.

FIELD WORK

The field work was planned for a two-week period in July between the end of the university term and the end of the school term. In the outcome approximately 90 per cent of the work was completed in this period. A small number of 'special' visits were done beforehand and the remaining 'mopping up' took a further four weeks.

In the sample were some three hundred dwellings which were inadequately defined. These were self-contained dwelling units with a single address but not identified by a separate number or letter at the time of the 1961 national census. They were identified in the sample list within the qualification 'any dwelling within', for example, 10 Town Place (any dwelling within). It was considered that unless these addresses were correctly sampled they provided a potential source of bias. If the dwelling chosen was always the most convenient, for example the ground-floor dwelling, or the one in which a person was present during the day, then the sample could be biased by the inclusion of an excess of elderly, disabled or other non-working persons.

To overcome this problem, these dwellings were enumerated by the permanent field-work staff in the week before the main operation started. Instructions were given that the number of dwellings within the address would be accurately determined, and one dwelling sampled by reference to a sheet of random numbers. If then, at this first visit, no answer was obtained from the selected dwelling within the address, as many further visits were made as were necessary to interview the residents.

The morning of the first day of the two-week period was used for instructing the students in the purposes of the study, some of the important underlying principles in sampling, study design and use of questionnaires, and in procedures for recording data. During the afternoon, each student was given a small number of addresses to visit and on return to base the results of his work and any other problems were discussed both individually and in groups with members of staff. At the end of the census there was general agreement among the students that, although they had been paid to undertake the work, it had proved one of the most enjoyable and illuminating ways of learning about the community.

The division of the study area into five working units required that some 1,100 dwellings were visited each day in the first week and again in the second week. To undertake this, a team of forty undergraduate medical and social science students worked during each day and an additional team of twenty students each evening. Every day each student was given approximately thirty addresses and was instructed to complete as many as possible. The work-load permitted repeat calls to be made at varying times throughout the day at any address at which no immediate contact was made. Each enumerator usually had between six and ten uncompleted addresses at the end of each day and these were reallocated to the students working in the evening. On the following day in each area, members of the permanent field-work team made any necessary follow-up visits.

One important aspect of the field work was the organization at the base for handling the mass of paper work involved in each day's operations. This involved a system for allocating each student's work-load for the day in as small a geographical area as possible, and for regrouping and reallocating the addresses still to be enumerated during the evening shift. To enable this to be done easily and quickly, as there was only half an hour between the day and evening shifts, each area was divided into eight sub-areas. By this system, and also by setting up a temporary base each day in the area to be surveyed, distances to be covered were kept to a minimum and the efficiency of the operation was improved.

In practice, the field work was not conducted to as rigid a pattern as the description of the broad outline might suggest. Considerable flexibility was retained, particularly in scheduling second visits. In addition, it was not always possible in the first weeks to contact the residents in some dwellings in multiple occupation. This meant that initial and second contacts in many dwellings were completed in the second and subsequent weeks.

However, some measure of the efficiency of the field work and of the methods used for recording the identifying data on each individual is given by the fact that at the end of the first week of field work approximately 3,000 enumeration forms were sent for the preparation of punch cards. A further 2,000 were dispatched at the end of the second week and the remainder followed in small batches over the succeeding four weeks. Coding of the questionnaires necessarily delayed their dispatch to the punch card operators but the last questionnaires were coded and delivered for punching with the last enumeration forms. Punching and verifying of each card was completed by a contracting agency within a week of the end of the field work.

Details of the size of sample and the outcome of the field work are shown in TABLE 2.

TABLE 2

NUMBERS IN RANDOM 1 IN 5 SAMPLE OF DWELLINGS IN SIX ELECTORAL WARDS OF NORTH LAMBETH WITH RESULTS OF FIELD WORK IN PRIVATE CENSUS

Random 1 in 5 sample of dwellings from 1961 national census lists .	5,640	
Random 1 in 5 sample of new hereditaments constructed since 1961 .	432	
TOTAL SAMPLE	6,072	
Dwellings known to be demolished before the start of field work .	326	
Dwellings found vacant during field work	200	
SAMPLE ELIGIBLE FOR ENUMERATION	NOS.	%
Total	5,546	100·00
Absolute refusals to co-operate	16	0·29
No contact made with occupants	13	0·23
Only partial information collected	18	0·32
Full information collected	5,499	99·16

An over-all response rate of full information collected from 99·2 per cent of dwellings was considered to be very satisfactory. A total population of 18,347 was enumerated.

An age–sex breakdown of the population is shown in TABLE 3 and a social class distribution of economically active or retired males in TABLE 4.

TABLE 3

AGE, SEX DISTRIBUTION OF ENUMERATED POPULATION

AGE	MALES		FEMALES	
	NOS.	%	NOS.	%
0–4	775	8·7	747	7·9
5–14	1,372	15·4	1,295	13·7
15–24	1,372	15·4	1,362	14·4
25–34	1,309	14·7	1,239	13·3
35–44	1,141	12·8	1,204	12·7
45–54	1,151	12·9	1,219	12·9
55–64	1,007	11·3	1,110	11·7
65+	779	8·8	1,265	13·4
ALL	8,906	100·0	9,441	100·0

It is possible to compare the distribution by age, sex, and social class of population enumerated by our private census with the population described by the one-in-ten sample census conducted by the General Register Office three months before, in April 1966. No statistically significant differences appear.

TABLE 4

PERCENTAGE DISTRIBUTION OF SOCIAL CLASS FOR ECONOMICALLY ACTIVE OR RETIRED MALES
(n = 6,759).

SOCIAL CLASS	%
I (professional)	1·97
II (managerial)	7·53
III (skilled)	53·63
IV (semi-skilled)	22·62
V (unskilled)	14·25

DATA PROCESSING

Using an I.B.M. 7090 electronic digital computer, five basic files of information were compiled on magnetic tapes:

1. An address code file. This contains the full postal address of each street, block of apartments, or named house to which a numerical address code was assigned. The file enables the coded addresses on the name cards and questionnaire cards to be printed out in full when required.

2. A master file compiled from the name cards and containing the information from the enumeration forms.

3. A master file compiled from the questionnaire cards and containing the information from the questionnaires.

4. A name, address, and data file compiled from the above three files and containing each sample address in full, followed by the name card and questionnaire card information for each person resident at the address. This file is held on six separate magnetic tapes, one for each electoral ward of the defined area. The format facilitates identification of individual persons by reducing computer time required for searching.

5. A copy of File 4 was created which is updated periodically in accordance with the information received on deaths, marriages, and migration in the enumerated population. This allows File 4 to remain untouched in order to represent the population at the time of census while making available an up-to-date file for sample identification purposes.

A print-out of the data as held on Files 2 and 4 is given in FIGURES 3 and 4 respectively.

However, before these data files could be finally established a checking procedure was undertaken. Apart from manual checking procedures, the computer was used to compare the data for each individual contained on the two punch cards, to apply limits to the codes used for recording questionnaire

```
46910050013551 7F964PATRICIA.ANNE        LARCOMBE              10000
4691006001354O0F903MAUD.MAY              HARRIS                10000
469101000035410F932OOROTHY               SPARROW               10000
4691010000354 11M927ALSTED               SPARROW               10000
4691010000354 12M961LEROY                SPARROW               10000
46910100003541 3F963MARCIA               SPARROW               10000
46910100003541 4F964VALERIE              SPARROW               10000
4691011000355 20M913HUGH                 ALSTON                10000
469101100035521F900ETHEL.LOUISE          ALSTON                10000
469101600035430F936MARION                HARRISON              10000
46910160003543 1F960ANN                  HARRISON              10000
469102000035440M934ANDREW.GREENLEES      NICOL                 10000
469102000035441F934JANET.ELIZABETH       NICOL                 10000
469102000035442M965ROBERT.HAROLD         NICOL                 10000
469102400035450F936ANNE                  HUGHES                10000
4691024000354 51M932WILLIAM              HUGHES                10000
4691024000354 52M964NEIL                 HUGHES                10000
469102400035453M961KEVIN                 HUGHES                10000
```

FIG. 3. Print-out from the master file of data from enumeration forms.

data and to check for incompatible combinations of codes. FIGURE 5 shows a specimen of the print-out of the check program showing how errors were identified for subsequent correction. Of the three examples, the first and third show discrepancies in the recording of year of birth on the two punch cards, and the second shows that the data as punched under hospital usage were incompatible.

```
2363 290 0   10  4      HUNTER HOUSE, ORSETT STREET, S.E.11.

         2363 290 0 49280 M 924   JOHN         RICHARDS
         2363 290 0 49281 F 929   JEAN         RICHARDS
         2363 290 0 49282 M 948   JOHN         RICHARDS
         2363 290 0 49283 F 950   MARY         RICHARDS
         2363 290 0 49284 M 951   KEVIN        RICHARDS
         2363 290 0 49285 M 954   JAMES        RICHARDS
         2363 290 0 49286 M 956   THOMAS       RICHARDS
         2363 290 0 49287 F 958   ALEXANDRA    RICHARDS
         2363 290 0 49288 F 960   GEORGINA     RICHARDS
         2363 290 0 49289 M 964   BARRY        RICHARDS

         2363 290 0 49280 1 924  1111112222 1 000000 2 050000 24237
         2363 290 0 49281 2 929  1111112222 1 000000 1 000000 25234
         2363 290 0 49282 1 949  1111112222 2 010000 2 010000 26147
         2363 290 0 49283 2 950  1111112222 1 000000 1 000000 24147
```

FIG. 4. Print-out from file containing address, identifying data, and other personal data.

Once the data files on magnetic tape had been established, computer output was required for clerical purposes, for the identification of stratified random samples and tabulations of analyses.

Output was required for the printing of two index cards per person to

I

```
(1014)  52 0 0  KENNINGTON ROAD, S.E.11.
HAS THE FOLLOWING INFORMATION WRONGLY CODED.    ••••••••••••••••••••••••••••••••••••••••••

YEAR OF BIRTH DISCREPANT,SERIAL NO IS ,  16492


(1014)  154 0 0  KENNINGTON ROAD, S.E.11.
HAS THE FOLLOWING INFORMATION WRONGLY CODED.    ••••••••••••••••••••••••••••••••••••••••••

MY SERIAL NUMBER IS   16560
THE FOLLOWING INFORMATION ARE IN ERROR.

IN-PATIENT HOSPITAL MISCODED  (COLS.38-43)


(1017)  117 0 0  LOLLARD STREET, S.E.11.
HAS THE FOLLOWING INFORMATION WRONGLY CODED.    ••••••••••••••••••••••••••••••••••••••••••

YEAR OF BIRTH DISCREPANT,SERIAL NO IS,  20121
```

FIG. 5. Specimen of print-out of check program.

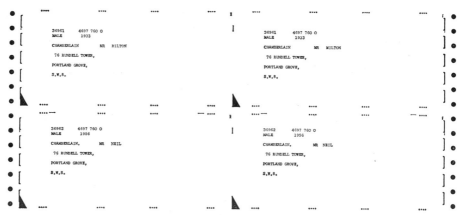

FIG. 6. Computer output on to index cards.

```
JANE PRICE.                                                      FEMALE    43   28390
     21 FENTIMAN ROAD,
        S.W.8.

DEREK PROOPS.                                                    MALE      27   28391
     29 FENTIMAN ROAD,
        S.W.8.

GEORGE MARSHALL.                                                 MALE      28   28392
     37 FENTIMAN ROAD,
        S.W.8.

FRANK HUNTER.                                                    MALE      40   28393
     43 FENTIMAN ROAD,
        S.W.8.

HILDA CAMPBELL.                                                  FEMALE    49   25860
     14 AIGBURTH MANSIONS,
        MOWLL STREET,
        S.W.9.
```

FIG. 7. Print-out of names and addresses of adults for the preparation of letters.

create manual card indexes to facilitate linkage and updating of records [FIG. 6], and for the printing of a list of persons enumerated [FIG. 7].

The list shown in FIGURE 7 was used for the preparation of letters sent to each address thanking respondents for co-operating in the study. This was undertaken not only to maintain goodwill, but also as a check on the performance of the field workers in correctly enumerating the given sample address. Both these procedures were completed within two months of ending the field work.

The first two studies following the census were planned to commence within four months of the end of the field work. For both these studies random samples were required. The first study was a check of the accuracy of reporting on hospital utilization. For this, a stratified random sample was drawn of persons who completed questionnaires, consisting of 1 in 20 of those reporting out-patient or casualty use only; 1 in 2 of those reporting in-patient use only; 1 in 5 of those reporting both types of use, and 1 in 50 of those reporting no hospital use. These sampling fractions were based on the total numbers of persons classified in these categories, as shown by analyses of the data obtained. A sample of 582 persons was identified. This sample was drawn and printed out by computer, as shown in FIGURE 8.

```
MYERS                 ,CECIL                    ( 1014 )   260 0   KENNINGTON ROAD, S.E.11.

SERIAL NUMBER    16490
SEX                  1
YEAR OF BIRTH     1893
SOCIAL CLASS         4
MARITAL STATUS       2
HSC                  7

OUT-PATIENT          2
OP - HOSPITAL 1     91
OP - HOSPITAL 2      0
OP - HOSPITAL 3      0

IN-PATIENT           2
IP - HOSPITAL 1     91
IP - HOSPITAL 2      0
IP - HOSPITAL 3      0
```

FIG. 8. Example of computer output of random sample selected for study of the accuracy of reporting hospital utilization.

The second study planned was a prevalence survey of chronic respiratory disease. For this, a sample was required of 1,500 males and females stratified by age, sex, and social class. The sample drawn and printed out by a computer was a systematic sample from a random start within each stratum. An example of the print-out of data obtained is given in FIGURE 9. For subsequent studies similar procedures have been used.

Perhaps the most obvious facility afforded by the use of the computer in such large-scale operations is the provision of detailed tabulations of data for the purposes of analysis. Using S.T.H. programs, tabulations of the data were obtained where not only the numbers of persons in any cell are displayed but also column and row totals, column and row percentages, column and row means and standard deviations, and chi-square calculations. As the program easily allowed for variation in the restrictions and for grouping of the characteristics under examination, and was able to perform either arithmetic or logical transformations of the data, exhaustive tabulations were quickly obtained. These provided both a clear presentation of the data and a basis for subsequent studies.

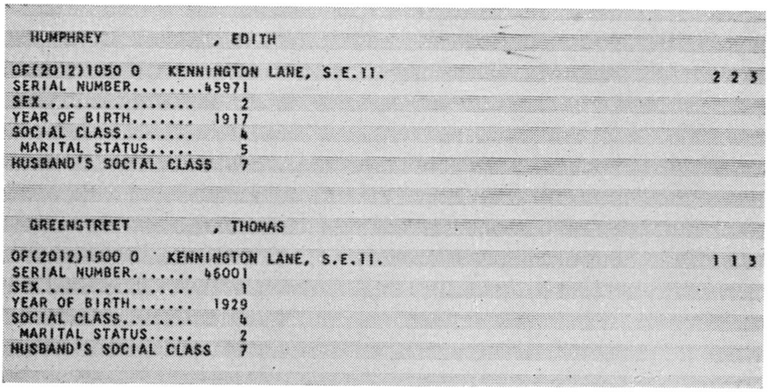

```
HUMPHREY              , EDITH

OF(2012)1050 0    KENNINGTON LANE, S.E.11.                2 2 3
SERIAL NUMBER........45971
SEX.................     2
YEAR OF BIRTH.......  1917
SOCIAL CLASS........     4
 MARITAL STATUS.....     5
HUSBAND'S SOCIAL CLASS   7

GREENSTREET           , THOMAS

OF(2012)1500 0    KENNINGTON LANE, S.E.11.                1 1 3
SERIAL NUMBER....... 46001
SEX.................     1
YEAR OF BIRTH.......  1929
SOCIAL CLASS........     4
 MARITAL STATUS.....     2
HUSBAND'S SOCIAL CLASS   7
```

FIG. 9. Example of computer output of random sample selected for cardiorespiratory disease study.

This description would be incomplete without some attempt to estimate the number of man-hours and computer hours in the procedures of data processing. It is estimated that the writing and testing of programs took 500 hours. However, this must be viewed not only as an investment in the immediate task but also as important investment for future studies. Programs were specifically written in such a way as to allow general applications in the future. Development occupied some 30 hours of I.B.M. 7090 computer time.

The procedures of data processing for the data collected involved six people for ten weeks. This includes time spent on the coding of questionnaires, checking and correction, which required a considerable amount of repunching of cards containing errors in the data. To obtain the desired computer output took some twelve hours of I.B.M. 7090 time and about eighteen hours of I.B.M. 1401 time. The time spent on the 1401 is understandable in view of the vast amount of output required in the form of listings. That spent on the 7090 appears considerable, but on the system employed includes time of tape manipulation and searching.

To conclude, the potentialities of the computer allow large studies to be planned and performed with the knowledge that the data collected can be quickly and accurately processed for the launching of further studies.

REFERENCES

BENNETT, A. E. (1966) Case selection in a London teaching hospital, *Med. Care*, **4**, 138.

GENERAL REGISTER OFFICE (1963) *Census of England and Wales 1961: County Report for London*, London, H.M.S.O.

MONTGOMERY, K. M. (1968) Out-patients of a London teaching hospital, *Brit. J. prev. soc. Med.*, **22**, 50.

10

COMPUTERS IN EPIDEMIOLOGY

F. J. MASSEY

RECENT ADVANCES IN COMPUTER USAGE

COMPUTERS are a relatively new tool. Although punch cards have been in use for a number of decades, the first practical electronic equipment—in the United States at least—dates from the middle 1940s. By the early 50s computers were widely used in certain industries, and since the late 50s their use has mushroomed. Today, university or research units which lack access to one or more computers are rare.

To most epidemiologists, however, the computer from, say, 1958–1963, was still a box (or a room) full of wires, for which extravagant promises were made, but which were typically out of order when they went to use them. Many must be familiar with the problems faced by the early computer users— the cards were mispunched or folded out of order, 'the room was too hot last night', etc. That 'system programmers changed the system last night', was, and still is, an unrebuttable reason for failure to get an answer. It would be impossible to pretend that these problems are now solved, but today the machine is at least much more likely to be a help than a hindrance.

One of the hardest problems for the researcher to face has, in the past, been the existence of a middleman, in the form of the programmer, the operator, etc., between himself and the computer results. This situation has gradually improved for several reasons. The first is the startling simplification of computer languages, so that if an investigator insists he can learn to program simple and even moderately difficult problems in a few days. Members of his staff can also be easily trained to do this. The second factor is the improved accessibility of computers, which means that in many installations a number of turn-arounds is possible in one day.[1]

The third factor contributing to the improvement of computer usage is the recognition that certain standard arrangements of data can be generalized to cover the majority of investigations in all fields of study. For example, suppose observations on an individual (or a city, an insect, etc.) are treated as a row of data, with repeated individuals giving repeated rows; the second

---

[1] Computer use involves both the submission of a problem and the achievement of a satisfactory output. The turn-around occurs when changes, additions, and/or corrections from the output are made and the problem is resubmitted.

variable in the row could then represent the age of a person in one study, the number of fatal accidents in another, the code for crooked wings in another, and so on. A further consideration of this approach will show that this matrix format is applicable to most epidemiological studies, and that, if we allow the number of observations per individual to vary, it would be difficult to imagine a study which would not partially fit into this format.

The problems of data processing in epidemiology are further lessened when one realizes that the mathematical analyses of the data used in perhaps 99 per cent of all applications are relatively few. (The really fierce problems in epidemiology are not data-processing orientated, but relate to the measurements, to case identification or location, to the establishment of reasonable denominators, etc.) Table construction—with corresponding percentages, chi-squares, means, standard deviations, correlation coefficients—probably accounts for the arithmetical techniques used in most articles in the *Journal of the American Medical Association*, the *Lancet*, and the *American Journal of Epidemiology*.[2] This technique, with the analysis of variance and covariance, multiple regression analysis, components-of-variance analysis, and a few non-parametric analyses, comprises all the methods of analysis currently used or needed by most research workers; in fact most investigators never employ all the techniques listed here.

With the recognition of the relatively few techniques required and of the value of standard data formats, almost all research-orientated computer facilities have now developed sets of package programs which an investigator without programming knowledge can use to obtain arithmetic processing of his data.

SOME LESS ROUTINE EXAMPLES OF COMPUTER USAGE

Discher, Massey, and Hallett (1969) report on a continuing surveillance and research programme where surveys are made with questionnaire data and X-ray findings recorded on punch cards. Digital recordings of ventilatory measurements are also made on magnetic tape. The cards and tape serve as input to a computer, which first analyses the time sequence of ventilatory values to compute such things as vital capacity and FEV, and then compares them with predicted values computed from height, age, etc. The computer prints these findings and prepares another magnetic tape with coded findings, name, address, etc. The second tape is used by a less sophisticated and cheaper computer to prepare typed letters which are mailed to participants, while copies are sent to their physicians.

Borun, Chapman, and Massey (1966) have recorded three lead vector

---

[2] It is important to stress here that statistics in the sense of statistical inference has been deliberately omitted, since it would be wise not to trust this to the computer. The latter should be used only for arithmetic, and not for deducing meanings and conclusions.

cardiogram signals on analogue magnetic tape. These are later digitized for analysis-comparison with standards, 'population' estimates, etc. Supplementary epidemiological data is collated and correlated with these findings in the computer.

The ability of the computer to prepare specified several-way frequency tables is well recognized. It is less well known that the speed of the large new machines makes it possible to have wholesale searches made of literally thousands of cross tabulations, the user's attention being called only to those of potential interest. This possibility raises serious questions of interpretation, in which the concept of the 'statistical level of significance' must be treated very cautiously. Inevitably, careful consideration will have to be given to the problem of deciding whether conclusions other than those for which the experiment was planned should be drawn from such analyses. The opinion of the author is that such findings should be considered tentative, and regarded only as hypotheses to be validated in other studies.

One important aspect of planning experiments and surveys is the careful allocation of resources, as the desired information should be obtained with the minimum of expense. Consideration must for example be given to the determination of necessary sample sizes[3] and to the specification of optimum and sequential programming of the steps of the experiment. Not infrequently, mathematical formulas for cost, time, and standard errors, etc., can be given, and the determination of parameters which minimize these functions is a classical numerical analysis problem for which computers are particularly valuable.

INDIVIDUAL AND LARGE-SCALE COMPUTERS

Computers today range in size from ones slightly larger than typewriters (e.g. those made by Wang, Olivetti, and Monroe) to those which fill a room (e.g. the larger of the I.B.M. 360 series and the C.D.C. 6000 series).

The 'size' of a computer has an important bearing on the speed of calculation, the amount and type of storage, the auxiliary hardware (types, discs, printers, etc.) and on the speed and convenience of input and output devices. If used efficiently, larger machines tend to cost less per result than small ones, but it takes a very large operation to keep a C.D.C. 6600 busy. Apart from simulation exercises, where millions of operations are repeated many times, the arithmetic speed of a computer is not of great importance to an epidemiologist. However, if a project involves a large amount of data with repeated analyses to be performed on the same data, convenient input is an important consideration. On medium to large computers the time used will cost several

---

[3] One reason for the scanty attention paid to the sample size determinations in textbooks is the difficulty of the related numerical problems.

dollars per minute, but in one minute many tables on hundreds of individuals can be produced.

All computers follow the same basic pattern: they accept 'input' information, follow programmed arithmetic or logical steps, and finally 'output' certain results.

A small computer will accept data from a keyboard, add it to a total, square it, and add to a second total, and then prepare to accept new data. If new data must be fed in manually, this is clearly inconvenient enough to consider using a larger machine with better input capability. On the other hand, if the data comes in small batches and is subjected only once to such arithmetic, the smaller equipment may be more than adequate. Medium and large models generally take input from punch cards and paper tape and produce output on a line-printer which can write several lines per second. Output in this form is, however, remote from the user.

Another important consideration related to size is access to the computer. If a large machine is overloaded with mandatory or higher priority work, or is badly staffed and unexpected problems constantly arise, there is a case for using more individual machines. With the advance of technology it will be possible for individuals or research units to have individual input and output consoles sharing time on a large basic computer with high speed and large storage. Again, with advancing technology, miniaturization is becoming possible, so that physically small computers with great computing power are becoming available. A choice between the two types of machine still remains, but the advantages of both are constantly improving.

COMMUNICATION WITH THE COMPUTER

In time-sharing situations, where the computer is not delayed by the hesitations of a single user, a typewriter console may be particularly useful. Instructions and data are then entered on the typewriter and are immediately transferred into the central computer for processing. Results may be given, by computer command, on the same typewriter used for input, or may be printed out for later distribution (a more remote process). The advantages of this system include the possibility of checking programs immediately, and, subject to the speed of the instrument, inspecting intermediate or final results as soon as they are produced. A major disadvantage is the difficulty of typing large quantities of data. However, data banks on tape or disc files which can be called into the computer without retyping are quite feasible. The introduction of a cathode ray tube enables results to be displayed more quickly and quietly, though there is a noticeable increase in cost. Points (or letters or numbers) are displayed in the C.R.T. at the command of the computer. A dialogue can then take place between the user and the machine, while the user types instructions or, if these are more limited, pushes a button;

the results required are then displayed on the tube. Figures and plots show quickly and clearly on the C.R.T., but a permanent copy of the results must also be obtained. In the future, we may expect to have printers, perhaps of an electrostatic nature, which combine the advantages of time, cost, and format. At present, however, permanent results must be printed out in the normal way.

FIGURES 10 and 11 are illustrations of results obtained by using a C.R.T. in this way.[4] In this calculation, the characteristics of population groups (for

EPIDEMIOLOGY VITAL STATISTICS GRAPHICS PROJECT

CAUSE OF DEATH LIBRARY

+	1	420.0 ASHD
+	2	420.1 ASHD INCL CHD
	3	410.0-419.9,420.2-434.4 OTHER HD
	4	440.0-443.0 HYP HD
	5	444-447 HYPERTENSION
	6	450 GEN ARTERIOSCLEROSIS
	7	451-468.3 OTHER CIRC DISEASE
	8	331 CEREB HEM
	9	332 CEREB THROMB
	10	330,333-334 OTHER CVA
	11	150-159 CA DIGESTIVE
	12	162-163 CA LUNG
	13	170 CA BREAST
	14	171-176 CA OTHER FEMALE
	15	177-179 CA MALE
	16	204 LEUKEMIA
	17	140-149,160-161,164-169,180-203,205 CA ALL OTHER
	18	480-493 INFLUENZA ETC.
	19	260 DIABETES MELLITUS
	20	581 CIRRHOSIS LIVER
	21	760-776 DISEASES EARLY INFANCY
	22	810-825,960 MOTOR VEHICLE ACCIDENTS
	23	830-959,961-964 OTHER ACCIDENTS
	24	980-985 HOMICIDE
	25	965-979 SUICIDE

FIG. 10. Cause of death library.

example, geographical or census tracts) had been stored on tape. Dynamic features of the population—deaths, births, illnesses, criminal acts, movement of home, etc.—were also available. Rates pertinent to selected population groups were required, either displayed on the tube immediately, or printed out within minutes. FIGURE 10, giving a cause of death library, appeared on the screen. Codes 1 and 2 (atherosclerotic heart disease) were selected, and after a 15-second search of the Los Angeles death records, the second table of rates [FIG. 11] appeared. The computer was then instructed to have both tables printed, as shown here.

With an attachment to convert a continuous signal into digital form, it is

[4] The figures are taken from the output of a graphic routine written by N. A. Eskind for the U.C.L.A. Epidemiology Division.

LOS ANGELES CITY DEATH RATES BY AGE, SEX, AND RACE
CAUSE OF DEATH= SUM 1, 2,

RESET END	PRINT	ALL			WHITE			NON-WHITE		
AGE		POPN	CASES	RATE	POPN	CASES	RATE	POPN	CASES	RATE
ALL	ALL	2477558	6898	278.4	2060576	6427	311.9	416982	470	112.7
	M	1196067	4127	345.0	992557	3838	386.7	203510	288	141.5
	F	1281491	2770	216.2	1068019	2589	242.4	213472	180	84.3
0- 4	ALL	249304	0	0.0	193209	0	0.0	56095	0	0.0
	M	126405	0	0.0	98226	0	0.0	28179	0	0.0
	F	122899	0	0.0	94983	0	0.0	27916	0	0.0
5- 9	ALL	221506	0	0.0	177281	0	0.0	44225	0	0.0
	M	112396	0	0.0	90220	0	0.0	22176	0	0.0
	F	109110	0	0.0	87061	0	0.0	22049	0	0.0
10-14	ALL	192470	0	0.0	158507	0	0.0	33963	0	0.0
	M	96904	0	0.0	80183	0	0.0	16721	0	0.0
	F	95566	0	0.0	78324	0	0.0	17242	0	0.0
15-19	ALL	147441	0	0.0	122653	0	0.0	24788	0	0.0
	M	70928	0	0.0	59363	0	0.0	11565	0	0.0
	F	76513	0	0.0	63290	0	0.0	13223	0	0.0
20-24	ALL	145875	1	0.7	116260	0	0.0	30615	0	0.0
	M	68384	1	1.5	54450	0	0.0	13934	0	0.0
	F	78491	0	0.0	61810	0	0.0	16681	0	0.0
25-29	ALL	164637	2	1.2	128663	1	0.8	35974	0	0.0
	M	83013	2	2.4	65213	0	0.0	17800	0	0.0
	F	81624	0	0.0	63450	0	0.0	18174	0	0.0
30-34	ALL	180715	14	7.7	145066	12	8.3	35649	2	5.6
	M	90007	13	14.4	72754	10	13.7	17253	1	5.8
	F	90708	1	1.1	72312	1	1.4	18396	0	0.0
35-39	ALL	193974	48	24.7	159002	39	24.5	34972	8	22.9
	M	94625	40	42.3	77468	33	42.6	17157	7	40.8
	F	99349	7	7.0	81534	5	7.4	17815	1	5.6
40-44	ALL	176191	103	61.3	147524	92	62.4	28667	16	55.8
	M	86089	92	106.9	72185	78	108.1	13904	13	93.5
	F	90102	16	17.8	75339	13	17.3	14763	3	20.3
45-49	ALL	164774	230	139.6	140140	200	142.7	24634	29	117.7
	M	80659	195	241.7	68518	174	253.9*	12151	21	172.8
	F	84105	34	40.4	71622	26	36.3	12483	7	56.1
50-54	ALL	144076	362	251.3	124680	324	259.9	19396	37	190.8
	M	69716	298	427.4	59890	270	450.8*	9826	27	274.8
	F	74360	63	84.7	64790	54	83.3	9570	8	83.6
55-59	ALL	130583	500	382.9	114368	452	395.2	16215	47	289.9
	M	62137	388	624.4	54115	359	663.4*	8022	28	349.0
	F	68446	111	162.2	60253	93	154.3	8193	18	219.7
60-64	ALL	110975	750	675.8	99820	693	694.2	11155	57	511.0
	M	50251	542	1078.6	44951	505	1123.4*	5300	36	579.2
	F	60724	208	342.5	54869	186	339.0	5855	20	341.6
65-69	ALL	95489	977	1023.2	86996	907	1047.6	8493	69	812.4
	M	41349	647	1554.7	37636	604	1604.8*	3713	42	1131.2
	F	54140	330	609.5	49360	303	613.9	4780	27	564.9
70-UP	ALL	144623	3898	2695.3	146407	3700	2527.2	12141	196	1614.4
	M	58663	1904	3245.7	57385	1793	3133.2*	5809	105	1824.8
	F	85960	1993	2318.5	89022	1902	2136.6	6332	90	1421.4

FIG. 11. Los Angeles city death rates by age, sex, and race.

possible to input electrocardiogram or respiration flow signals directly into a computer for analysis.

In the type of calculations described above, the computer enables traditional arithmetic to be performed faster or more extensively. Moreover, there are other situations where the contribution of the computer is unique, as in, for example, modelling, data banks, and teaching.

MODELLING AND SIMULATION

Almost without exception, deterministic and probability mathematical models of epidemics have resulted in equations which could not be handled explicitly, except in the most trivial situations. In other words, the study of a realistic epidemic process could not be carried out mathematically. With the arithmetic power of large computers it is now possible to study some models numerically, though work in this field has only just started.

It is now also possible to set up a population and use a chance device (for example, random numbers generated in the computer) to determine the state of the population at the next time period. This is repeated, and the progress of the simulated epidemic is displayed on the cathode ray tube. The same process is performed over and over again until probable results are determined, or until visual characteristics of the epidemic curve are seen and noted. This type of simulation (without the cathode ray tube output) of a probability model of an epidemic, where movement of participants was allowed, is described by Bailey (1967). In his model he was able to consider the effect of changing contact probabilities on an outcome such as the number of new cases per area unit.

CENTRAL LIBRARIES

Certain airlines have a reservation service in which flight information, including seat reservations, are filed in a computer memory. Telephone inquiry from any one of hundreds of service points gives information on seat availability, and if new reservations or cancellations are made, the file is updated accordingly. In the same way, a number of large health facilities or community health planning groups are now studying suitable methods of collecting and collating data which will allow computers to assist in community planning, to retrieve information in emergencies, or to facilitate demographic studies.

Although the system is not yet in commercial production, the Bell Telephone Laboratories have developed a *Picturephone*; input is read in by a push button, the signal is transmitted over telephone wires to a remote computer, and the output is returned to a cathode ray screen. Similar units have currently been developed which have permanent special wiring for the cathode ray units, although a typewriter unit does transmit over telephone wires. In Los Angeles an ambulance is being equipped to transmit electrocardiogram signals to a hospital; it is clearly the next step to transmit these signals to a computer.

In view of these developments, it is easy to imagine that in the near future a field epidemiologist will be able to dial his findings to a central unit on a cordless telephone.[5] He could possibly also use a portable blood analyser

---

[5] A wristwatch phone has been used in a United States comic strip for several years. It is clearly within the scope of present technology to have a remote computer console which could be carried on the front seat of a car and which could communicate with the computer over a car phone.

which would feed measurements to the computer, diagnostic findings being reported back within seconds. It is not unreasonable to expect that a search of records for similar disease reports could be made without operator intervention, and that, if the situation warranted, officials could be alerted. In a similar way it is possible to imagine a computer stopping traffic in smog alerts, stopping sales of particular drugs when samples (automatically obtained) showed impurities or age effects, or calling for an immunization programme when an epidemic of a serious disease appeared to be developing. This last possibility is, however, remote, since the models for epidemic predictions are at present insufficiently developed for use in dealing with practical problems. It is, in fact, very doubtful whether the stochastic models for the epidemic process will be sensitive enough to change in parameters, so that such predictions can be made from observations on an epidemic already in progress.

We can, however, at least expect such central libraries to have connections with most public and private health workers; reports of many diseases will immediately be filed so that, where diagnosis is possible, up to the minute morbidity information could be available and assembled. Practitioners would also be able to identify by computer inquiry whether symptoms observed in one patient were observed in others.

TRAINING

One method of teaching is to expose the student to the conditions of a dynamic problem and let him react. This has been simulated in epidemiology by, for example, telephone conversations where an outbreak of a particular disease is reported. The student asks questions as to signs or symptoms, requests information as to possible sources of infection, or directs that preventive or curative action should be taken. The teacher then responds appropriately both to the student's answers and to the training objective.

In 'business games' computers have been introduced into this type of learning experience: opposing teams decide on business actions (buy, sell, stockpile, spend money on research, and so on), the computer uses an economic model to predict results, and these are in turn used by the teams to make further decisions. It should be stressed that, whether the model describes the real world correctly or not, the participants in the game obtain a real experience, bringing to bear the operational dynamics relating to action, time, and money.

It is quite clear that such computer learning games will become available and will be used in epidemiology. Factors relating to cost of health officer decisions (in money, time, public relationships, or more illness) as well as population characteristics, could, for example, be considered. The information could be derived from books, or obtained by querying the computer.

Alternatively, some information could be given by the computer, with some choice left to the player. A health report, for example, of a case of a strange but unidentified disease could be generated and a response expected. Possible responses range from noting, but taking no action on, the report, requesting further information about the case, asking the central files if any other such symptoms have been reported and 'sending' an investigator to take laboratory measurements. The particular response given would in turn lead the computer to generate one of several possible consequences.

As in the business game, time is the important factor: asking questions over the phone gives a certain amount of information quickly, reference to books may involve more time, and sending a field investigator would involve even more. Two time scales would be needed, one the real time of the player, and the other that simulated for the investigation. The field investigator's report back would be phased appropriately by the computer, and interactions would of course occur, so that secondary health reports might come in before the report of the field worker.

REFERENCES

BAILEY, N. T. J. (1967) The simulation of stochastic epidemics in two dimensions, *Proc. Fifth Berkeley Symp. Math. Statist. Probab.*, **4**, 237.
BORUN, E. R., CHAPMAN, J. M., and MASSEY, F. J. (1966) Electrocardiographic data recorded with Frank Leads, *Amer. J. Cardiol.*, **18**, 656.
DISCHER, D. P., MASSEY, F. J., and HALLETT, W. J. (1969) Quality evaluation and control methods in computer-assisted screening, *Arch. environm. Hlth*, **19**, 323.

PART VI

ANALYSIS

11

MODELS FOR INFECTIOUS DISEASES

H. V. MUHSAM

INTRODUCTION

MODEL building is one of the most powerful means of gaining insight into the internal structure of an imperfectly known phenomenon or process. To fulfil this function a model must obviously be more than a replica on a different scale (like the model of a building), and it is certainly neither an object nor a pattern to be reproduced by imitation (like an artist's model), or regarded as a standard or an ideal worth striving for. These are some of the meanings of the word 'model' in everyday language. But when we talk of models in the physical and biological sciences, we do refer to a replica of a phenomenon or, more often, a process, though for the most part neither differences in scale nor those in material between the real world and the model play any role: the model belongs, in general, to a completely different universe. We may construct, for example, physical models of social structures and geometric models of physical entities. The mathematical models of epidemic and demographic processes with which we are concerned here are also typical examples.

A warning should be expressed against the danger of confusing mathematical representations and models. A mathematical formulation of a phenomenon can be called a 'model' only if it is able to describe, express, perhaps explain, and often test a hypothesis regarding its internal functioning; otherwise it is a mere mathematical representation. Similarly, the 'model' of, say, an internal combustion engine serves mainly to demonstrate the working of such a motor.

Therefore, all the constants, variables, parameters, and operators which appear in the mathematical formulae of the model have a definite meaning in terms of the observed, observable, assumed, or imputed attributes of the object to be represented by the model. Moreover, these mathematical formulae often serve to bridge the gap between various observed quantities, or between *a priori* assumptions and observed facts. A mathematical model can be considered as promising if it permits one to reproduce or to predict observable quantities in a satisfactory way, obviously without introducing them explicitly or implicitly into it. But the main criterion for the quality of a model is its success in supplying a fair picture of the circumstances, forces,

K

or determinants which operate in reality. It should, however, be admitted that these circumstances, forces, and determinants may actually not be known; their image in the frame of the model is often their whole essence.

AN EXAMPLE

In most of the mathematical models with which we are concerned here, a population of a given number, N, of individuals is classified into k classes, such as the three (that is, in this example $k = 3$) categories, 'susceptible', 'infective', and 'immune' with respect to some infectious disease. The state of the population is then fully described by the k quantities N_1, N_2 . . . , N_i . . . N_k; the course of the events, for example the process of the epidemic, reflects itself in the changes which occur in the numbers N_i, in our case in the numbers of susceptibles, infectives, and immunes in the population. A graphical representation of the course of the epidemic, showing the changes which occur in the numbers of each class (susceptibles, infectives, immunes) may be very useful—but this is not what should be called a model. The graphical representation may show very clearly how the reservoir of susceptibles is emptied slowly into the class of infectives which in turn is ultimately exhausted by transfers into the category of immunes; this is not a 'model', because it 'explains' very little of the processes involved.

What is the kind of information, explanation, prediction, etc., which we expect from a model and which is not supplied by a graphical representation or other mathematical description? Let us consider, first of all, what interests us in an epidemic, restricting ourselves to looking at the figures N_i as functions of time. Then we shall see what has to be fed into the model as building material, what else is needed as fuel to make it work, and finally, what it is able to produce.

The following is an illustrative list—neither comprehensive nor selective— of items which might be of interest in the example of the epidemiological situation under consideration and which the model is expected to explain or to predict:

1. The presence of very few infective cases in a large susceptible population often does not trigger an epidemic; there is some kind of threshold involved.

2. The number of new infective cases is, at the beginning of an epidemic, relatively small, it then increases slowly at first and later rapidly, and finally tapers off. Outbreak and tapering off are not necessarily of symmetric shape.

3. Some epidemics spread rapidly, others slowly.

4. Not all susceptibles are necessarily infected before the epidemic subsides.

The main building materials for our model are the following facts, assumptions and restrictions: the population of N individuals is classified into k classes with N_i ($i = 1, 2, \ldots, k$) individuals in each class, so that $N_1 + N_2 + \ldots + N_k = N$; the state of the population at any time t is fully described by the quantities N_i; individuals can pass from one class to another only according to a set of rules; in our example all individuals are initially susceptible—they may become infective, and infectives eventually all become immune. The architect's work consists now in choosing the functions Φ_i which permit one to compute the quantities N_i at any time on the basis of the factors or parameters α_i, determining the course of events— $N_i = \Phi_i(\alpha_i, N_j, t)$, where $j = 1, 2, \ldots, i, \ldots k$. The selection of these functions is guided by two principles: known or assumed mechanisms involved in the phenomenon which is the object of the model, and mathematical manageability. The former may relate either to the behaviour of individuals or to mass action—but this differentiation is not always clear. Nevertheless, we speak often of micromodels as against macromodels and refer then to this aspect of model building. It may be mentioned that micromodels are, in general, probabilistic or, as it is called in this context, stochastic, while macromodels are typically deterministic.

Let us come back now to our consideration, how to build our model. First, the universe of factors, circumstances and conditions which are known or assumed to affect the course of events, is divided into two parts: those which are considered as constant, negligible, or not interesting, in the frame of the proposed analysis, and those which should be taken into consideration. Thus, in most epidemiological models, the course of events, that is, the numbers of susceptibles, infectives, and immunes existing, at any moment, in the population, as well as any changes occurring in these numbers, are assumed to be fully determined by the corresponding numbers immediately before that moment, together with some measure of the contagiousness of the disease under consideration. As a contrast, in a model of human fertility, the transition of a woman from the status of pregnant to that of non-pregnant depends not only on her status in the previous month but also on her status during each of the last nine months (or even more): obviously, if a woman had been pregnant for between one and eight months, her position in the following month would differ from that of a woman who had been pregnant for the nine consecutive months.

Thus, in our simple epidemiological model all the $N_i(t)$ are fully determined by the $N_j(t - \Delta t)$ where $j = 1, 2, \ldots, i, \ldots k$ and Δt is a short time interval. Thus $N_i(t) = \Phi(N_j(t - \Delta t))$.

The next step in building the model consists of selecting the functions Φ_i which permit the computing of numbers which are of interest, on the basis of all the data which have been assumed to affect these numbers. In our simple epidemiological example, we accept that any change in the number of susceptibles, N_1, is due to the infection of susceptibles by infectives, N_2; the volume of this change is assumed to be proportional to the numbers of both susceptibles and infectives. This proportionality can be justified in many different ways: for example, it seems reasonable to assume that, if a certain number of infections occur in a group of susceptibles of given size, twice as many infections may be expected to occur in a group of twice that size, *ceteris paribus*; similarly if, with a given number of infectives in a population a certain number of infections do occur, doubling the number of infectives would be expected to double the number of new infections. These two assumptions of proportionality are not the only possible ones. A different set of assumptions has recently been proposed by Severo (1967) and will be discussed below. In this example these assumptions are the main input into the model.

This input can be translated into the language of mathematics by the differential equation

$$\frac{dN_1}{dt} = -\beta N_1 N_2,$$

where the parameter β now makes its appearance. It stems from the fact that we assumed 'a certain number' of infections, and that 'twice as many' would occur without specifying the 'certain' number.

This is one of the advantages of the language of mathematics: it does not permit any vagueness. But this remark has little to do with model building in general, although it is of relevance to all mathematical models. From the aspect of model building, we have here the second main input: it is item 3 of the above short list of interesting facts which is now fed into the model. Indeed β is the rate of infectiveness or the 'infection rate' of the disease: it is the number of new cases per susceptible and per infective in the population per time unit. This model assumes infectiveness to be constant for any epidemic, that is, for all infectives, all susceptibles, and throughout the course of the epidemic. This is obviously a simplification of the model, which is introduced mainly for the sake of manageability and which cannot always be justified.

If we remember that all additions to the number of infectives arise from withdrawals from the population of susceptibles, and that withdrawals from the number of infectives equal increases in the number of immunes, both being proportional to the number of infectives, we obtain two more differential equations, namely

$$\frac{dN_2}{dt} = \beta N_1 N_2 - \gamma N_2 \quad \text{and} \quad \frac{dN_3}{dt} = \gamma N_2,$$

where γ has a meaning vaguely similar to that of β: it is the 'removal rate'.

The mathematical solution of these three simultaneous equations supplies the desired functions Φ_i: it is our model. Unfortunately, the solution cannot be expressed by means of simple algebra; to some extent, our model violates the requirement of manageability. But in the eye of the mathematician, the set of differential equations is perfectly equivalent with its solution. Thus the set of differential equations can already be considered to be our 'model'.

Does this model fit reality? All three remaining items of interest on the above list (item 3 having already been accounted for) are 'predicted' by the model:

1. A relation exists between the infectiveness of the epidemic, the removal rate and the size of the population which determines the conditions for the outbreak of an epidemic, when a very small reservoir of infection is introduced. Only if the infection rate is higher than N times the removal rate, that is, $\beta/\gamma > N$, is an epidemic triggered in the presence of a mere trace of infection. This is the so-called threshold theorem. When a sizeable number of infectives is introduced into a population, the epidemic always spreads at least to some extent. But if the infection rate is not higher than a fraction $1/(N - A)$ of the removal rate (A being the number of infectives introduced into the population), the spread of the disease consists only of the phase of subsidence of the epidemic.

2. The typical course of an epidemic, that is, the peaked 'epidemic curve', showing the number of infections per time unit, is very well reproduced by the model, including its lack of symmetry.

3. The 'intensity' of the epidemic, that is, the proportion of the susceptibles who contract the disease, may take all values between 0 and 100 per cent. It is determined by the ratio between infection and removal rates. Unfortunately, its value cannot be expressed in a simple arithmetic manner.

This is the description of a model—in fact Kendall's (1956) deterministic epidemic model. It is built on the few very simple assumptions which are set out above; the fuel, which makes it run, consists of the two parameters, infection and removal rates. The model produces predictions regarding three important characteristics of an epidemic, and if empirical observations of the characters of an epidemic are consistent with the predictions supplied by the model, the model can be considered as valid.

It furthermore 'explains' why it is not any isolated case of an infectious disease that necessarily triggers an epidemic: there is a threshold effect. It also explains why it is not always all susceptibles who contract the disease: the threshold conditions may be reached during the course of the epidemic long before all susceptibles have been infected, and the epidemic then tapers off without reaching all susceptibles.

But the main contribution of the model to the understanding of the epidemic lies in the corroboration it supplies for the assumptions which led to the basic differential equations. These assumptions imply that the danger of contracting the disease increases with the number of infectives, that is, the risk of an infection depends on the number of infectives. In other words, the infection can be considered as a chance event, with constant probability measured, somehow, by the parameter β. The probability concept was not explicitly introduced here, but in some other models it fulfils the function of the basic assumption.

A CLASSIFICATION OF MODELS

The model of an epidemic which we have just described is deterministic. In such a model, the course of events is fully determined by the initial conditions, the values of the parameters which are accepted and, obviously, the structure of the model.

That this is somehow unrealistic is most easily seen through the micro-approach. Any new infection is, from the point of view of the epidemiologist and from that of the man in the street, a 'chance event' in the sense that, under given circumstances, a susceptible runs only a certain risk of being infected; he is never necessarily infected. There is, in other words, a certain probability that any susceptible will be infected—and this does not happen with certainty to any given person nor to a given number of persons; the number of those who escape infection is obviously also affected by chance. Thus, so-called 'stochastic models' may perhaps supply a more realistic picture of the actual events.

At the same time, we may notice that the numbers N_1 in which we are interested do not change continuously, but in steps, of exactly one at least. Moreover, we are not often interested in the state of the population at any time, but only at certain moments which do not follow each other continuously, such as successive generations (for example, in studies of population genetics). Fortunately, stochastic models work very well with discrete variables (such as numbers of susceptibles, etc.) or in discrete time.

Joshi (1967) has recently proposed a classification of models of the type with which we are concerned here, by distinguishing not only between those that are deterministic and stochastic but primarily whether the variables which are studied (in our case N_1) are considered as continuous or discrete, which similarly applies to time. Thus Joshi distinguishes four main types of models:

1. Continuous Variables, Continuous Time

The model discussed above as our main example belongs to this type. It has recently been generalized on the basis that the number of susceptibles who become infective in a given time interval are not simply proportional to the numbers of susceptibles and infectives (Severo, 1967[1]). It was proposed

[1] Severo actually discussed a 'continuous time-discrete variable' model.

to assume that this number was determined by the numbers of susceptibles (N_1) and infectives (N_2) according to the function of the type $\beta N_1^{1-b} N_2^a$, where β is, as above, the infection rate, while a is called the 'infective power' and b the 'safety-in-number power'. An appropriate choice of a permits one to include certain epidemics in the model even when the number of infections remains relatively small ($a < 1$), as well as epidemics whose spread increases much more quickly than the number of infectives ($a > 1$). At the same time, the generalization permits one to account for the possibility of some kind of safety provided by the existence of a large number of susceptibles (b relatively large), as well as for the case where the number of new infections is almost completely independent of the number of susceptibles ($b \cong 1$).

Other generalizations of the basic model become necessary, to fit the course of an epidemic which is caused by a parasite needing, in addition to the human host, another host or carrier to complete its life-cycle. Well-known examples are malaria and schistosomiasis.

A model of the malaria epidemic, which takes into account the fact that two hosts are involved, has been developed by Macdonald (1957) and Macdonald, Cuellar, and Fall (1968). It is obvious that when the role of the mosquito in the transmission of malaria is explicitly introduced, the simple model of a probability of infection which is proportional to the number of infectives does not suffice: somehow, the number of mosquitoes must, at least, be introduced. In fact, it is not only the number of mosquitoes in the area but a whole list of variables and conditions which apparently affect the spread or the abatement of the epidemic. Macdonald explicitly introduces the following parameters:

1. The anopheline density in relation to man.
2. The number of men bitten by, at least, one mosquito in a day.
3. The proportion of anophelines with sporozoites in their glands, which are actually infective.
4. The probability of a mosquito surviving one whole day.
5. The time taken for completion of the extrinsic cycle.
6. The proportion of the human population receiving inocula in one day.
7. The proportion of the human population actually infective.
8. The recovery rate, i.e. the proportion of the infectives who revert to non-infective, per day.
9. The incubation interval.

The model permits the determination of 'threshold' conditions not as a simple function of infection and recovery rates, but in terms of all nine parameters. This is highly valuable information for planning the struggle against the disease: it becomes possible to weigh the effects of different approaches to the eradication of the disease one against another, taking both cost and efficiency into consideration. Such different approaches may consist in attempts to reduce, for example, the density of mosquitoes per man, the probability of a mosquito surviving one whole day, the number of bites, the proportion of infectives in the human population, etc. And the efficiency of any measure depends on the form in which it appears in the 'threshold' condition, at least whenever it is the aim of the campaign to keep condition beneath the threshold.

A similar model has been built for schistosomiasis (Macdonald, 1965). Obviously, other factors play their role here, such as:

1. A contamination factor, measuring the number of eggs introduced into the water, which depends on the prevalence of the disease and the level of sanitation.

2. A snail factor, measuring the chances of a miracidium coming into contact with a snail. This depends on the density of the snail population.

3. An exposure factor, measuring the chances of a cercaria finding a human host. Here human behaviour patterns play the decisive role.

4. A longevity factor, which reflects mainly the total number of eggs laid by a parasite.

Macdonald's model introduces these factors explicitly, in a set of equations similar to those of our previous example, but in this case he considers also the chances of a male parasite meeting a female in the human host. Here, the assumption of continuity of the variables can obviously not be maintained. The main results are of the same type as in the model for malaria: they permit prediction of the effect of different measures which can be taken in the struggle against the disease. Macdonald shows that, in practice, it is impossible to eradicate the disease by sanitation only. A campaign consisting of treatment of the affected population, which reduces the contamination factors, together with as much snail control and reduction of the exposure factor as can be put easily into practice, can be expected to bring the disease under control after being maintained for about 75 years. Only the eradication of snails and radical control of exposure promise much quicker success.

2. *Continuous Time, Discrete Variables*

In discrete-variables models, account is taken of the fact that the numbers of individuals in each of our categories may change only in steps of at least one person. In epidemiology, this type of model, with continuous time, was developed in detail by Bailey (1953). In the original form of the model the removal of infectives into the category of 'immunes' (or kept in isolation, deceased, etc.) is disregarded; this simplification seemed necessary in view of mathematical difficulties which otherwise arise.

As with these assumptions of discreteness we are dealing with stochastic models, we can no longer consider directly the number of persons moving from the category of susceptibles to that of infectives: we can only speculate about the probability of a susceptible becoming infective. This probability is assumed to be proportional to the number of infectives and susceptibles in the population, as in the equivalent assumption about the number in the deterministic model.

The results to which this approach can be expected to lead are obviously only the probabilities that the population will be, at a given time, in any of the different possible states, the probabilities of all possible courses of events, as well as those of all different possible outcomes of the epidemic. These are certainly more realistic, though perhaps less useful, results than those of deterministic models: it is obvious that the course of an epidemic is not predetermined but depends on many chance events.

However, the most likely, the expected (in the sense of 'expected value') or average course of an epidemic is of special interest. It is easily proved mathematically that it does not differ fundamentally from that obtained by the corresponding deterministic model.

A demographic example of the continuous-time, discrete-variables type is a model used by Perrin and Sheps (1964) to study human reproduction. Here we are faced by five classes in our population of women:

   i. non-pregnant, fecundable
   ii. pregnant
   iii. post partum sterile after abortion
   iv. post partum sterile after stillbirth (no lactation)
   v. post partum sterile after live birth

Transitions are permissible only from category i to ii; from ii to iii, iv and v; and from iii, iv, and v to i.

When suitable assumptions are made about the probabilities of the permissible transitions, the following interesting characteristics of the population can be determined:

1. The distribution of women by the number of times they make, during a certain period, the transition from state i to state ii or from ii to v, etc.

2. The distribution of women by the duration of their stay in each of the states, for example i.

3. The probability of a birth occurring, in any given month, to a woman.

4. The recurrence time, that is, the time it takes, on an average, (or the distribution of women by the length of this time) to return to the same stage, for example stage v (post partum sterile after live birth).

This model obviously applies only to a cohort, or otherwise defined population, of women who are characterized by a uniform level of fertility, which is assumed not to change as a consequence of ageing, of successive pregnancies, or of their outcome.

This model may find useful applications also in epidemiology, when an infectious state is followed by a state of immunity of limited duration, after which the patient again becomes susceptible.

3. *Continuous Variables, Discrete Time*

This is the type of model which is widely used in demography, in the study of both 'natural' growth of populations and migratory movements. Often these models are deterministic, and in the field of natural growth they can be used to prove Lotka's stable population theorem.

In this approach to Lotka's theory, the population is observed at discrete points in time, for example, once in five years. It is then assumed that the number of persons of given age is, at any time, a certain proportion—according to the respective survivorship rate—of the population of an appropriate younger age at the time of the previous observation. Moreover, the number of persons in the lowest age group is the sum of numbers (of births, less infant deaths occurring in the meantime) which stand in given proportions to certain categories of the population (women of reproductive age) at the previous observation.

It should be stressed that we are not concerned here with a population of constant number N; on the contrary, the behaviour of N at successive observations is the main point of interest. It is, indeed, one of Lotka's assertions that the rate of increase of N becomes constant, as do the proportions of persons in the various age groups. This assertion is easily proved if formulated through this model, in view of some well-known theorems of Markovian processes.

For the building of a model of this type for the analysis of migrations (Muhsam, 1963), it is assumed that given proportions of the population of any class, which now represents a geographical area, are found at each consecutive point in time, in the same class (non-migrants) and in each of the other classes (migrants from one area to another). The total population remains, in pure migration models, constant. Thus, the model permits one to prove that if the population sticks to its migratory behaviour for a long enough time, its geographical distribution becomes constant. These ultimate, constant proportions of the population to be found in each area arise only from the model and do not exist in reality: they are an expression, an image, or even a measure of the actual migratory behaviour of the population, and have been claimed to have more socioeconomic relevance than the migratory movements themselves.

If natural increase or external migrations are also incorporated in the model (Muhsam, 1964) and show geographical differentials, the model permits differentiation between what are sometimes called 'demographic' and 'economic' migrations. By 'demographic' migration we understand those internal migration streams which merely compensate for differential natural growth and the unequilibrated influx of immigrants into some of the regions. 'Economic migrations' are the response of the population to socioeconomic differences between the various geographical areas. Such a differentiation—between demographic and economic migrations—obviously does not exist in the mind of a migrant, nor does it permit classification of individual migratory moves. It is again only an artifact of the model. In this sense, the main contribution of the model owes its whole existence to the model; but it permits important progress in the understanding of, and theory-formation in, this complicated field of internal migrations.

Thomlinson (1961) has developed a stochastic model for problems of the same type. In such a model, the proportion of persons who actually migrate is replaced by the probability that a person will migrate.

4. *Discrete Variable, Discrete Time*

The Reed–Frost formulation of the mathematical theory of epidemics is the best-known example of this type of model. The discreteness of the variables reflects, as usual, the fact that the number of individuals of any category changes in steps of at least one; and the discreteness of time implies that the state of the population is observed only at certain, generally equidistant, points of time. In the Reed–Frost theory, points of time separated by an interval of the latent period of the epidemic disease are taken into consideration. Thus, so to speak, successive 'waves' of the epidemic, separated by the incubation period of new cases, are the subject of this model.

The main advantage of the 'discrete-time' approach lies in the fact that, within a given lapse of time which is not infinitesimal, the chances of one susceptible having contact with one, two, three, etc., infectives gains real meaning; obviously a susceptible who has more than one appropriate contact with an infective, contracts the disease only once. Thus, the effect of the number of infectives on the spread of the disease in the population is different here from what it would have been according to the continuous-time model. This becomes especially important in small populations such as a family, a children's home, etc. Indeed, the Reed–Frost model applies fairly well to the situation in such small groups. Empirical data on epidemics observed in communities of limited size fit fairly well with the model when an appropriate probability of infection is selected. Thus, the danger of infection in a family can be compared with that in a children's home, a village, etc., on the basis of the observed course of an epidemic in such groups.

The classic Reed–Frost model has been generalized in many directions, for example, by Bailey (1953) and Abbey (1952). However, it is not the purpose of this survey to describe or even give a list of such modifications; the following may, however, serve as an example.

It is assumed, in an approach which was also presented by Bailey (1955), that the probability of infection varies from one susceptible to another. If we now study the spread of infection in families of different size, the chances of catching a first infection no longer depend directly on the number of members of the family, but also on their proneness to contract the disease. In families of given size, say three members, each member may have a different chance of infection: P_1, P_2 and P_3. If each family is assumed to contain one member characterized by P_1 (the father), another by P_2 (the mother) and a third by P_3 (the child), these three probabilities can be estimated from the relative frequencies of the different 'chains' of infection, without considering the personal roles of father, mother, and child in the chain. There are indeed seven different possible 'chains' in a family of three: if all members ultimately contract the disease, one initial case may be followed by two cases at the second stage ('chain'; 1–2) or by one at the second and another at the third (1–1–1). There may be two initial cases (2–1) or three initial cases (3). Furthermore, two members (with two possible chains: 1–1 and 2), and finally, one member only of the family may contract the disease. Each of these chains has a different probability of occurrence; and in any empirical study, the seven observed frequencies may permit one to estimate the three basic probabilities. Thus, we can test the hypothesis that each family of three is made up of persons who belong each to a different class with respect to the probability of infection.

Other modifications affect different aspects of the Reed–Frost model, and other models differ in many aspects from those which we used as examples. But it was not our intention to discuss all models nor could we possibly list them, together with their modifications, variations and generalizations. Surveys of this type were prepared by Dietz (1967) and Gurland (1964), to mention only two recent publications.

But at least one aspect which this survey has not dealt with at all certainly deserves more attention than some of those on which we dwell at comparative length: this is the spread of an epidemic from its source over a wide area. Several recent authors have started to develop means of tackling this aspect; at least Neyman and Scott (1964), Kendall (1965), and Bailey (1967) should be mentioned here. Its importance lies in the fact that the geographical spread of epidemics is perhaps the most frequently observed aspect and, at the same time, the most neglected one in analyses. On the other hand, to restrict an epidemic to the limited area in which it made its first appearance is one of the main endeavours of epidemiological policy. But theory and models have not yet been able to contribute much to practical work in this field.

CONCLUSION

Several models have been described, all of which have actually been proved to be suitable for fitting to empirical data. Attempts have been made to show the contribution of models to understanding of the forces which act in the development of the phenomena which they describe, and to planning the control of epidemics. At the same time, some hints could be given on the flexibility of models: many may be easily amended, to account for specifications and details which differ from one case to another or were even disregarded in the main formulation of the model. Some models may even be applied in different branches of science.

It should, however, be stressed that this last aspect—the applicability of the same model in various processes and phenomena, sometimes from different scientific disciplines—should not be interpreted as a 'proof' of the 'truth' of the model. No model has any reality in itself: it is never more than a contraption which may help to understand and to interpret empirical data, or a device for forming hypotheses and testing them, regarding the forces which affect observed courses of events.

However, from the point of view of both the theoretician and the practitioner, a model certainly presents a clearer picture of the essence of the phenomena which they observe than the observations themselves.

REFERENCES

ABBEY, H. (1952) An examination of the Reed–Frost Theory of epidemics, *Hum. Biol.*, **24**, 201.

BAILEY, N. T. J. (1953) A simple stochastic process, *Biometrika*, **37**, 193.

BAILEY, N. T. J. (1955) Some problems in the statistical analysis of epidemic data, *J. roy. statist. Soc.*, Ser. B, **17**, 35.

BAILEY, N. T. J. (1967) The simulation of stochastic epidemics in two dimensions, *Proc. Fifth Berkeley Symp. Math. Statist. Probab.*, **4**, 237.

DIETZ, K. (1967) Epidemics and rumours, a survey, *J. roy. statist. Soc.*, Ser. A, **130**, 505.

GURLAND, J., ed. (1964) *Stochastic models in Medicine and Biology*, University of Wisconsin, Wis.

JOSHI, D. D. (1967) Stochastic models utilised in demography, *World Population Conference, 1965*, Vol. III, New York, p. 227.

KENDALL, D. G. (1956) Deterministic and stochastic epidemics in closed populations, *Proc. Third Berkeley Symp. Math. Statist. Probab.*, **4**, 140.

KENDALL, D. G. (1965) Mathematical models of the spread of infection, in *Mathematics and Computer Science in Biology and Medicine*, London, H.M.S.O., p. 213.

MACDONALD, G. (1957) *The Epidemiology and Control of Malaria*, London.

MACDONALD, G. (1965) The dynamics of helminth infections with special reference to schistosomes, *Trans. roy. Soc. trop. Med. Hyg.*, **59**, 489.

MACDONALD, G., CUELLAR, C. B., and FALL, C. V. (1968) The dynamics of malaria, *Bull. Wld Hlth Org.*, **38**, 743.

MUHSAM, H. V. (1963) Toward a formal theory of internal migrations, *International Population Conference 1961*, Vol. 1, New York, p. 333.

MUHSAM, H. V. (1964) The isolation of the effect of differential natural growth on internal migrations, *Population Conference 1963*, Ottawa, p. 423.

NEYMAN, J., and SCOTT, E. (1964) A stochastic model of epidemics, in *Stochastic Models in Medicine and Biology*, ed. Gurland, J., University of Wisconsin, Wis., p. 45.

PERRIN, E. B., and SHEPS, M. C. (1964) Human reproduction, a stochastic process, *Bull Int. Inst. Statistics.*, **40**, 1067.

SEVERO, N. C. (1967) *Generalisation of Some Stochastic Epidemic Models*, 36th session of the International Statistical Institute, Sydney, Paper 2/90.

THOMLINSON, R. (1961) A model for migration analysis, *J. Amer. statist. Ass.*, **61**, 675.

12

MULTIVARIATE ANALYSIS

A. E. Maxwell

INTRODUCTION

THIS chapter is divided for simplicity into two parts. Part I deals with problems of discrimination which arise when the statistician is presented with scores, or ratings, on several variables for samples drawn from supposedly different populations of patients and already allocated to diagnostic categories, for example, paranoids, schizophrenics, anxiety states, psychopaths, etc. The task here is primarily to see to what extent the categories are justified in the light of the relatively objective data supplied by the scores or ratings or, conversely, to demonstrate that additional variables are necessary if the initial categories are to be retained. Several multivariate statistical methods, already relatively well known, are employed in the examination of some real data to illustrate how such procedures can throw light on the problems raised. The topics discussed are Profile Analysis, Discriminant Function or Canonical Variate Analysis, and Multivariate Analysis of Variance.

The number and variety of multivariate techniques now available to the applied statistician is already great, and no attempt will be made here to give an exhaustive account of them. Instead, a few of the techniques found useful for dealing with recurrent problems will be briefly described.

Part II of the chapter deals with problems which have been somewhat neglected by statisticians in the past but which are currently receiving wide attention. They are variously considered under such titles as 'numerical taxonomy', 'clustering', or 'clumping'. Psychiatrists in general are unhappy about the objectivity of current diagnostic practice, and are appealing to the statistician for help in clarifying the situation. Hence there is a growing tendency to present him with scores or ratings on a set of variables for a heterogeneous sample of patients which, it is suspected, has been drawn from a composite population, in the hope that, on the basis of the data, he will be able to separate the patients into relatively homogeneous subsamples, representative of a number of recognizable subpopulations. Two possible statistical procedures for achieving this are illustrated and critically examined. The chapter ends with a list of references which, though far from complete, is fairly representative.

I. PROBLEMS IN THE DISCRIMINATION OF PSYCHIATRIC PATIENTS

PROFILE ANALYSIS

An investigator frequently has scores, or ratings, on several variables for each patient in a number of samples of patients. It will be assumed that the variables are normally distributed (or can be transformed to achieve normality), and that the samples are drawn at random from different psychiatric categories of patients. The problem is to decide whether, on the evidence available, the categories are recognizably distinct. The profiles for the samples are obtained by plotting the mean scores of the variables, as in FIGURE 12. They are then compared. The attraction of the method is that

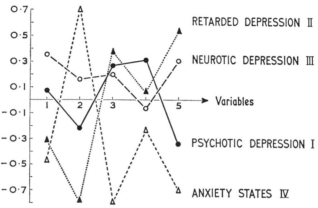

FIG. 12. Profiles for four diagnostic categories.

it provides a good visual picture of the data; but appearances can be deceptive if variation within samples is considerable, consequently a statistical assessment of the data is desirable.

If the variables were uncorrelated, the investigator might be advised to perform a simple analysis of variance on group means separately for each variable. If significant differences were found and these differences were sufficiently large to be of *clinical importance*, then he might be able to answer his question satisfactorily in this way. But in general the variables will be fairly highly correlated. Patients who have 'thought disorder' are frequently also 'hallucinated'; anxious patients are often also obsessional; and so on. Consequently, some more elaborate form of analysis, which takes possible correlations between variables into account, is likely to give a more satisfactory answer. It has, too, to be remembered that the psychiatric classification of patients is seldom, if ever, based on the presence or intensity of a single symptom, but rather on a syndrome of symptoms not all of which may be present in the case of any single patient in a given category.

To illustrate the method of profile analysis it will be helpful to consider a real example. A psychiatrist interested in 'affective conditions' had data on five variables for a sample of patients from each of the four following diagnostic categories:

Category	Sample size
I Psychotic depression	13
II Retarded depression	13
III Neurotic depression	32
IV Anxiety states	16

The five variables were (a) worrying; (b) anxiety; (c) depression; (d) obsessional traits and ideas of reference, etc.; and (e) irritability, loss of interest, etc. He wanted to find out whether, on the evidence available, the four diagnostic categories used were justified, or whether some of the categories might well be combined.

Each variable consisted of a rating scale on which the patient was allotted a score for the symptom concerned. Since these scales had different ranges it was decided, for the purpose of comparing the group profiles, to transform the data so as to equate the scales. This was done by calculating the over-all mean, $\bar{X}$, and within-group variance, s^2, for each variable and performing the transformation

$$Y_{ij} = (X_{ij} - \bar{X})/s$$

where X_{ij} is the score for the ith patient in the jth category for the variable in question. The procedure assumes that the variance in the subpopulations (categories) for each variable are homogeneous and that the samples are sufficiently large to get stable estimates of them. The mean scores for the four categories on the five variables after transformation are shown in TABLE 5 and are plotted in FIGURE 12.

TABLE 5

MEAN SCORES FOR CATEGORIES I TO IV ON VARIABLES a TO e

CATEGORIES	VARIABLES					OVER-ALL MEANS
	a	b	c	d	e	
I	0·0448	−0·2862	0·2484	0·3108	−0·3434	−0·0051
II	−0·3048	−0·7888	0·3706	0·0651	0·5694	−0·0177
III	0·3420	0·1288	0·1414	−0·0086	0·2478	0·1703
IV	−0·4728	0·6158	−0·7858	−0·2881	−0·6792	−0·3220

L

The questions generally asked in profile analysis are:

1. Are the groups on the same level, i.e. do the groups arise from populations having the same over-all group means?
2. Do the groups arise from populations having parallel group profiles?

These questions can be answered to a good approximation by a two-way analysis of variance, with interaction (Box, 1949; Greenhouse and Geisser, 1959). An analysis of the data for categories I and III is given in TABLE 6.

TABLE 6
TWO-WAY ANALYSIS OF VARIANCE FOR PATIENTS
IN CATEGORIES I AND III

SOURCE OF VARIATION	D.F.	MEAN SQUARES	F-RATIO
Between Categories (C) . . .	1	1·420	—
Between Variables (V) . . .	4	0·414	—
Interaction (CV) . . .	4	1·317	1·86 N.S.
Patients within Categories . . .	43	2·839	—
Residual	172	0·708	—

From the analysis in TABLE 6 the question of whether the groups are at the same level can be tested by the F-ratio 1·420/2·839, with 1 and 43 degrees of freedom. In this instance the test would not lead one to discard the null hypothesis. The question of whether the two profiles are parallel would be tested by the ratio of the 'interaction' and 'residual' means squares, but difficulties now arise. It is known that this test is valid only in cases where the variates have equal variances and are independent, or at least equally correlated in pairs for all categories. If the assumptions of independence or of equal correlations are not met then the degrees of freedom for both numerator and denominator have to be fractionally reduced. The procedure is described by Box (1949) and by Greenhouse and Geisser (1959). The fraction required in this example is 0·821, which reduces the degrees of freedom of 4 and 172 to 3·3 and 141·2 respectively. With these values and an F-ratio of 1·86 the interaction term is found not to be significant. Hence, there are inadequate grounds for assuming that the profiles for categories I and III are not parallel. The conclusion reached is that the variables employed give insufficient evidence for differentiating between neurotic depressives and psychotic depressives.

If the data for all four categories are included in a single analysis of variance, similar to that shown in TABLE 6, significant differences between 'levels' $(P<0·01)$ and a significant interaction effect $(P<0·01)$ are found. But it is best to analyse the profiles two at a time, for interpretation of the results is then straightforward.

If a more exact analysis than that given in TABLE 6 were required a full multivariate analysis could be carried out (Morrison, 1967). For two categories of patients the data, assuming p variates, can be set out as in TABLE 7 in which x_{ijk} stands for the score of the ith patient on the jth variable in the kth category.

TABLE 7

SCORES FOR PATIENTS IN TWO CATEGORIES FOR p VARIABLES

CATEGORIES			PATIENTS	VARIABLES $x_1 \ldots x_j \ldots x_p$		
	I		1	x_{111}	x_{1j1}	x_{1p1}
			.	.	.	.
			.	.	.	.
			.	.	.	.
			n_1	x_{n11}	x_{nj1}	x_{np1}
Vector of means	.	.	.	$\bar{x}._{11}$	$\bar{x}._{j1}$	$\bar{x}._{p1}$
	ll		1	x_{112}	x_{1j2}	x_{1p2}
			.	.	.	.
			.	.	.	.
			.	.	.	.
			n_2	x_{n12}	x_{nj2}	x_{np2}
Vector of means	.	.	.	$\bar{x}._{12}$	$\bar{x}._{j2}$	$\bar{x}._{p2}$
Vector of mean differences, $\mathbf{d}'$	.			$(\bar{x}._{11} - \bar{x}._{12}) \ldots (\bar{x}._{p1} - \bar{x}._{p2})$		

If the data are normally distributed and the variance–covariance matrices within the subpopulations are homogeneous the equality of the two vectors of means can be tested using Hotelling's T^2 statistic. Briefly the procedure is as follows. Let the corrected sums of squares and cross products for the two categories be represented by the two $p \times p$ matrices $\mathbf{W}_1$ and $\mathbf{W}_2$. Then an estimate of the within categories variance–covariance matrix is given by $\mathbf{S}$, where

$$\mathbf{S} = (\mathbf{W}_1 + \mathbf{W}_2)/(n_1 + n_2 - 2). \qquad (1)$$

The T^2 statistic is

$$T^2 = \frac{n_1 n_2}{n_1 + n_2} \mathbf{d}'\mathbf{S}^{-1}\mathbf{d}, \qquad (2)$$

where $\mathbf{d}'$ is the vector of mean differences shown in TABLE 7. The quantity

$$F = \frac{T^2(n_1 + n_2 - p - 1)}{p(n_1 + n_2 - 2)} \qquad (3)$$

is then referred to the F-distribution with p and $(n_1 + n_2 - p - 1)$ degrees of freedom. If a significant result is obtained, then at least one pair of mean differences $(\bar{x}._{j1} - \bar{x}._{j2})$ is significantly different from zero. (It should be noted that this test is not equivalent to the test between 'levels' given in TABLE 6.)

Of greater interest in the present context is the use of the T^2 statistic for testing whether the group profiles are parallel. Here the problem is one of testing whether the $1 \times (p - 1)$ vector of means

$$(\bar{x}._{11} - \bar{x}._{21}), (\bar{x}._{21} - \bar{x}._{31}), \ldots (\bar{x}._{(p-1)1} - \bar{x}._{p1})$$

for the first category differs from the $1 \times (p - 1)$ vector of means

$$(\bar{x}._{12} - \bar{x}._{22}), (\bar{x}._{22} - \bar{x}._{32}), \ldots (\bar{x}._{(p-1)2} - \bar{x}._{p2})$$

for the second category. In this instance W_1 and W_2 are matrices of order $(p - 1)$, where the $(p - 1)$ new variates are obtained from those in TABLE 7 by subtracting the second column of scores from the first, the third from the second, etc. A new vector of mean differences d'_1 and a new S - matrix, S_1, is now obtained. T^2 will become

$$T^2 = \frac{n_1 n_2}{n_1 + n_2} d'_1 S_1^{-1} d_1, \tag{4}$$

and the quantity

$$\frac{T^2(n_1 + n_2 - p)}{(p - 1)(n_1 + n_2 - z)} \tag{5}$$

can now be referred to the F-distribution with $(p - 1)$ and $(n_1 + n_2 - p)$ degrees of freedom. If a significant result is obtained the differences which contribute to it can be isolated (Morrison, 1967, p. 125).

If more than two categories were concerned then Hotelling's T^2 test could not be employed and multivariate analysis of variance would be required to test the equality of the mean vectors. Briefly, the procedure is as follows. If there are k categories, a $p \times p$ matrix, B, of corrected sums of squares and cross-products between category means is obtained. Within-category corrected sums of squares and cross-products matrices, W_1, W_2, $\ldots$, W_k are also obtained and are pooled into a total 'within' matrix W, where

$$W = W_1 + W_2 + \ldots + W_k.$$

Several test statistics for testing the equality of the mean vectors have been suggested (Morrison, 1967, Ch. 5) of which the Wilks' criterion, $\Lambda = |W|/|B + W|$, and the Hotelling statistic, trace $(B W^{-1})$, are the best known. But the validity of these tests depends on $N = (n_1 + n_2 \ldots + n_k)$ being large. For relatively small N the best procedure seems to be one given by

Heck (1960), in which the largest latent root of the matrix $\mathbf{B}\,\mathbf{W}^{-1}$ is referred to a set of specially prepared charts.

By telescoping the p variables into a set of $(p - 1)$ differences between pairs, as in the second paragraph above, the profiles for more than two groups can also be simultaneously compared, using Heck's test.

DISCRIMINANT FUNCTION OR CANONICAL VARIATE ANALYSIS

Since the publication of Fisher's and Mahalanobis' (1936) papers, interest in multivariate analysis of discriminance has been steadily growing. Useful reviews are those by Wishart (1955) and Bartlett (1965) while modern textbooks on multivariate analysis (for example, Morrison, 1967; Rao, 1952) treat the subject in considerable detail.

In this chapter an approach commonly used for appraising a prior allocation of patients to diagnostic categories will be described and some examples given. The method derives from Rao's generalization to several groups of Fisher's discriminant function method for two groups.

As in the case of profile analysis it will be assumed that within a broad class of psychiatric patients k relatively distinct subclasses exist. Samples from the subclasses are available with scores on each of p variables, x_1 to x_p. The purpose of the analysis is to set up a weighted function $f(x)$ of the variables

$$f(x) = w_1 x_1 + w_2 x_2 + \ldots + w_p x_p, \tag{6}$$

such that the F-ratio for the weighted mean scores for the samples in a one-way analysis of variance is maximized. The problem can be formulated concisely in matrix algebra. Let $\mathbf{B}$ be the 'between-groups' $p \times p$ matrix of sums of squares and cross-products of the x-scores about their respective means, and let $\mathbf{W}$ be the corresponding 'within-groups' matrix. Now if the $p \times 1$ column of weights is represented by the vector $\mathbf{w}$ (with transpose $\mathbf{w}'$) the problem is one of finding that set (or sets) of weights which maximizes the expression

$$\lambda = (\mathbf{w}'\mathbf{B}\mathbf{w})/(\mathbf{w}'\mathbf{W}\mathbf{w}). \tag{7}$$

In this expression both the numerator and the denominator are scalar quantities. Moreover, if the total sample size is N the degrees of freedom for 'between' and 'within' groups are $(k - 1)$ and $(N - k)$ respectively. Hence

$$\lambda = \frac{k - 1}{N - k}\, F. \tag{8}$$

Maximizing λ is thus seen to be equivalent to maximizing the F-ratio between groups, and so of maximizing the difference between group means. The assumptions made in this procedure are that the x-scores for the respective groups are multivariate normal and have equal variance–covariance matrices.

On differentiating expression (7) with respect to the $\mathbf{w}$'s, rearranging and equating to zero, the equations

$$(\mathbf{W}^{-1}\mathbf{B} - \lambda\mathbf{I})\mathbf{w} = \mathbf{O} \tag{9}$$

are obtained, where $\mathbf{I}$ is the unit diagonal matrix. The solution of equations (9) involves finding the latent roots, λ_i, and corresponding latent vectors $\mathbf{w}_i$ of the asymmetric matrix $\mathbf{W}^{-1}\mathbf{B}$. The number of latent roots possible will depend on the rank of this matrix. It can be shown to be equal to p or $(k - 1)$ whichever is the smaller. It follows that when only two groups are concerned only one set of weights and consequently only one discriminant function or canonical variate results. In other cases more than one set of independent weights may result. The number of functions which is then considered depends on the number of latent roots that is significant; the relevant test has been given by Bartlett (1947).

Since rapid and powerful methods of finding the latent roots and vectors of symmetric matrices on computers are available, it is advisable first to put the matrix $\mathbf{W}^{-1}\mathbf{B}$ into symmetric form. Let $\mathbf{T}$ be a lower triangular matrix with positive diagonal elements, such that $\mathbf{TT'} = \mathbf{W}$. Then the matrix $\mathbf{T}^{-1}\mathbf{BT'}^{-1}$ has the same latent roots as $\mathbf{W}^{-1}\mathbf{B}$. Moreover, if $\mathbf{u}_r$ is the latent vector of $\mathbf{T}^{-1}\mathbf{BT'}^{-1}$ corresponding to the rth latent root then the corresponding latent vector of $\mathbf{W}^{-1}\mathbf{B}$ is $\mathbf{w}_r = \mathbf{T'}^{-1}\mathbf{u}_r$.

Bartlett's test for the significance of the latent roots is a chi-square test in which

$$X^2 = [n - \tfrac{1}{2}(p + k)] \log_e (1 + \lambda_j), \tag{10}$$

with $(p + k - 2_j)$ degrees of freedom. Here λ_j refers to the jth latent root; $n = N - 1$, where N is the total number of patients involved; p is the number of variables and k the number of groups or categories.

CANONICAL VARIATE ANALYSIS—AN EXAMPLE

A canonical variate analysis was carried out for the four samples of patients considered in the profile analysis. The latent roots of the matrix $\mathbf{W}^{-1}\mathbf{B}$ are given in TABLE 8, together with the tests of their significance.

The fact that only the first latent root is significant and is numerically much larger than the other two indicates that variation between the four categories can be accounted for adequately along a single dimension. The weights corresponding to the first latent root, scaled so that the variance of the weighted scores is 0·9259, and the correlations between each of the variables and the first canonical variate also appear in TABLE 8.

The weights can now be placed in equation (6) above and a score for each patient on the canonical variate obtained. These scores are invariant in the sense that if the scores on one of the original variables are multiplied (divided) by a constant the corresponding canonical variate weight is divided (multiplied) by the same constant, hence the canonical variate score for a patient is unaltered. It follows that, in general, a canonical variate should not be interpreted in terms of the relative sizes of the weights unless the

TABLE 8

LATENT ROOTS AND FIRST CANONICAL VARIATE WEIGHTS OF BW^{-1}. CORRELATIONS OF FIVE VARIABLES WITH THE CANONICAL VARIATE

LATENT ROOTS	D.F.	CHI-SQUARE	SIGNIFICANCE
1. 0·92587	7	44·89	Sig.
2. 0·12127	5	7·84	Non-Sig.
3. 0·10480	3	6·83	Non-Sig.

VARIABLE (X)	WEIGHTS FOR FIRST CANONICAL VARIATE	CORRELATIONS BETWEEN VARIABLES AND CANONICAL VARIATE
1	0·388	0·137
2	0·793	0·606
3	−0·738	−0·481
4	−0·175	−0·091
5	−0·194	−0·295

variables all have the same metric. For purposes of interpretation it is thus desirable that a computer program gives the correlations between the observed variables and the canonical variates. In our example the results show that the canonical variate correlates positively with 'anxiety' and negatively with 'depression', the other correlations being of rather negligible magnitude. The variate thus seems to represent a dimension running from 'anxiety' at the positive pole to 'depression' at the negative pole.

The mean scores and their standard errors for the several samples on the variate are given in TABLE 9.

TABLE 9

MEAN SCORES ON FIRST CANONICAL VARIATE

CATEGORY	MEAN CANONICAL VARIATE SCORE	STANDARD ERROR OF MEAN
I Psychotic depressives . . .	−0·2513	0·2669 (13)
II Retarded depressives . . .	−0·6112	0·2669 (13)
III Neurotic depressives . . .	0·1332	0·1701 (32)
IV Anxiety states . . .	1·2468	0·2406 (16)

The smaller size of the standard error for neurotic depressives is simply a reflection of the larger sample size ($N = 32$) in this category. If required, differences between means can now be compared, but it is clear that categories II and IV are farthest apart. More valuable information is obtained by plotting the distributions of the patients' scores and examining them. This is done in FIGURE 13.

Here it is seen that the neurotic depressives are a very mixed bag; that the retarded depressives and psychotic depressives are very similar, and that apart from a few outliers (probably misclassified patients) in the psychotic depressive

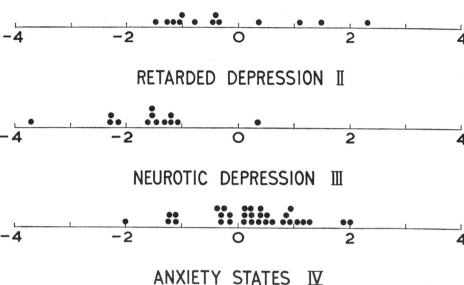

FIG. 13. Canonical variate scores for four categories.

category, this category and the retarded depressives overlap very little with the anxiety states. We need not dwell on interpretation here, but the analysis is clearly a great improvement on the profile analysis.

Interpretation of the results of a canonical variate analysis increases in complexity when more than one of the latent roots of $\mathbf{W}^{-1}\mathbf{B}$ is significant. For two significant latent roots the data can still be plotted, taking axes at right-angles to represent the two canonical variates obtained. This is legitimate since the canonical variates are orthogonal. The space can then be partitioned among the groups so as to minimize misclassifications [FIG. 14]. For further interesting examples see Healy (1965) and Slater (1960).

For more than two canonical variates the problem is more difficult. In some early work (Rao and Slater, 1949), procedures are described for calculating the likelihood that a patient, drawn arbitrarily from a composite population, came from one of the subpopulations within it. The patient is then allocated to the subpopulation for which his likelihood is greatest.

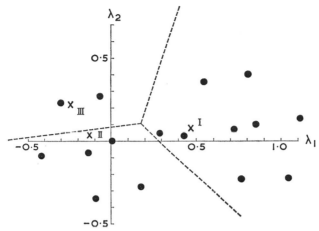

FIG. 14. Mean scores for categories I, II, and III plotted as X's. Pattern scores plotted as dots.

But the procedures have shortcomings especially when the prior probabilities of a patient belonging to one or other of the subpopulations are unknown, and when the variance–covariance matrices have to be estimated from rather limited data. More recently the problems which arise have been ably discussed from a Bayesian viewpoint by Geisser (1964), while Hills (1966) discussed in detail 'the problem of choosing allocation rules and assessing their errors of misallocation' when two subpopulations are involved and the data are qualitative.

DICHOTOMOUS DATA

Although there is an increasing tendency for psychiatrists to use rating scales for assessing the severity of patients' symptoms, data do occur in which only the presence (generally scored '1') or absence (scored '0') of symptoms are recorded. Experience has shown that when sample sizes are reasonably large such data can, with advantage, be analysed by the same methods as were used with continuous variables.

In TABLE 10 data are given for three random samples from the following diagnostic categories (Maxwell, 1961):

I Schizophrenics ($n_1 = 244$)
II Manic depressives ($n_2 = 279$)
III Neurotics ($n_3 = 117$)

for the four dichotomously scored symptoms: (*a*) anxious; (*b*) suspicious; (*c*) thought disorder; and (*d*) delusions.

A canonical variate analysis, similar to that described earlier, was performed on these data. The matrix $\mathbf{W}^{-1}\mathbf{B}$ gave two significant latent roots,

TABLE 10

SYMPTOM PATTERNS AND THEIR FREQUENCY OF
OCCURRENCE IN THREE PSYCHIATRIC DIAGNOSTIC
GROUPS (I TO III)

FREQUENCY OF OCCURRENCE OF SYMPTOM PATTERNS IN GROUPS

PATTERN NUMBER	*a*	*b*	*c*	*d*	I	II	III	λ_1	λ_2
1	0	0	0	0	38	69	6	0	0
2	0	0	0	1	4	36	0	−0·10	−0·34
3	0	0	1	0	29	0	0	0·86	0·12
4	0	0	1	1	9	0	0	0·76	−0·22
5	0	1	0	0	22	8	1	0·29	0·04
6	0	1	0	1	5	9	0	0·19	−0·30
7	0	1	1	0	35	0	0	1·15	0·16
8	0	1	1	1	8	2	0	1·06	−0·18
9	1	0	0	0	14	80	92	−0·33	0·25
10	1	0	0	1	3	45	3	−0·43	−0·09
11	1	0	1	0	11	1	0	−0·53	0·37
12	1	0	1	1	2	2	0	0·43	0·03
13	1	1	0	0	9	10	14	−0·04	0·29
14	1	1	0	1	6	16	1	−0·14	−0·05
15	1	1	1	0	19	0	0	−0·82	0·41
16	1	1	1	1	10	1	0	0·72	0·07
		TOTAL			224	279	117		

namely $\lambda_1 = 0\cdot9533$ and $\lambda_2 = 0\cdot2009$, ($P < \cdot001$ in each case). The corresponding latent vectors were

$$\mathbf{w}'_1 = (-0\cdot33 \quad 0\cdot29 \quad 0\cdot86 \quad -0\cdot10), \text{ and}$$
$$\mathbf{w}'_2 = (\quad 0\cdot25 \quad 0\cdot04 \quad 0\cdot12 \quad -0\cdot34),$$

and the mean scores on the two canonical variates for the three categories were found to be:

Categories				Mean Scores on Canonical Variates	
				(1)	(2)
I Schizophrenics	.	.	.	0·490	0·098
II Manic depressives		.	.	−0·157	0·013
III Neurotics	.	.	.	−0·274	0·229

These mean scores are plotted as X's in FIGURE 14. A score for each patient on each canonical variate could also be calculated and plotted, and the variate space could then be partitioned between the categories so as to minimize the number of misclassifications. The scores for each answer pattern are shown in TABLE 10 columns (λ_1) and (λ_2) and are plotted in FIGURE 14.

The above example has an obvious defect because the four symptoms used are not adequate for discriminating effectively between categories II and III. As is clear from TABLE 10, 80 patients out of the 279 manic depressives and 92 out of the 117 neurotics have the same symptom pattern, namely (1 0 0 0); but the example shows that the method is useful.

II. PROBLEMS IN THE CLASSIFICATION OF PSYCHIATRIC PATIENTS

INTRODUCTION

In my experience, psychiatrists seldom if ever use the statistician's discriminant functions or decision rules when classifying patients into diagnostic categories. In the first place, the number of variables employed by the statistician is seldom adequate to cover all facets of abnormal behaviour, and in the second place, his models frequently (as in Part I) are based on samples of patients already allocated to diagnostic categories about which there is some dispute. It would thus appear that the primary value of the methods of discrimination, discussed in Part I, lies in the light they throw on the adequacy of objective measures to reflect the clinician's diagnostic practices, and on his need to be more explicit about the information he uses when making a diagnosis. Undoubtedly there is a growing desire among psychiatrists to come to better agreement about the diagnostic categories they use and any assistance the statistician can offer is likely to be welcome.

CLUSTERING

One problem on which advice is frequently sought is that of 'clustering'. Here, as already noted, the statistician is presented with a sample of patients from some composite population, say *psychotic patients* or *neurotic patients*, and on the basis of certain observations on these he is asked to subdivide them into a number of reasonably distinct clusters. The psychiatrist wishes to see the extent to which the statistician's subdivisions agree with his own independent allocation of the patients to diagnostic categories.

Now the word 'cluster' is difficult to define precisely, though intuitively its meaning is fairly clear. If a sample of patients can be subdivided into clusters it is implied that a patient in one cluster has a symptomatology more similar to other patients in that cluster than to patients in a different cluster.

One way of deriving clusters is to calculate 'coefficients of similarity', or other similar measures, between all pairs of patients and then to scan the results. For symptoms which have been recorded as present (1) or absent (0) the results for each pair of patients can be set out in a fourfold table as follows:

$$
\begin{array}{c|cc}
 & \multicolumn{2}{c}{\text{Patient } j} \\
 & 1 & 0 \\
\hline
\text{Patient } i \quad \begin{array}{c} 1 \\ 0 \end{array} & \begin{array}{c} a \\ c \end{array} & \begin{array}{c} b \\ d \end{array}
\end{array}
\qquad (a + b + c + d = N),
$$

where a, b, c, and d represent the frequency of matches and mismatches (1,1), (1,0), (0,1) and (0,0) respectively. Several different formulae for calculating similarity coefficients have been suggested (Sneath and Sokal, 1963; Joyce and Channon, 1966); examples are $(a + d)/N$ and $a/(a + b + c)$. The main difficulty in deciding on a coefficient seems to hinge on the question of whether or not to include d. Clearly if d were large compared with a, b, and c, the coefficient of similarity would tend also to be large but it would reflect 'non-information' rather than 'positive' information. The problem requires investigation but will not be discussed further here.

Several methods of automatic classification have been proposed (Sneath and Sokal, 1963), and a program widely used in the United Kingdom is one by Mr. J. Gower called CLASP, written for the Orion Computer at Rothamsted. For this program the data may be in the form of dichotomies, but continuous data can also be dealt with. Gower employs a similarity coefficient S_{ij} between the ith and jth object (person) which is defined so as to lie in the range 0 to 1. The results of each test (t) for objects i and j are compared one by one and assigned a *score* s_{ij} which lies between 0 and 1 and a *count* n_{ij} which is 1 if the test gives a valid comparison and 0 otherwise. Then

$$S_{ij} = \Sigma s_{ij}/\Sigma n_{ij}$$

where the summation extends over all tests. For dichotomous data scoring is as follows:

	s_{ij}	n_{ij}
t_i or t_j unknown	0	0
$t_i = t_j = 0$	0	0
$t_i = t_j = 1$	1	1
$\left.\begin{array}{l} t_i = 1,\ t_j = 0 \\ t_i = 0,\ t_j = 1 \end{array}\right\}$	0	1

Variants of this scoring method are used for qualitative and quantitative data.

For a given level of similarity L a grouping $G(L)$ of the set of objects can be defined such that every object belongs to a group and no object belongs to more than one group. CLASP will set up 'single linked' groups in which every member of the Group G_i is similar to some other member of the group at a level greater than L, but similar to all non-members of G_i at a level less than or equal to L. These groups cannot be further subdivided. L is initially set to a maximum level and is decreased by a constant amount at each stage, continuing until there is only a single group, or zero level is reached.

Other writers on classification have used the chi-square statistic as a measure of association between tests, or have employed measures of 'information' in the Shannon–Weaver sense, based on fourfold contingency tables. A useful summary of these methods is given by MacNaughton–Smith (1965) and further details will be found in Williams and Lambert (1959, 1960).

DISTANCE FUNCTIONS AND DISPERSION ANALYSIS

Since data of the form depicted in TABLE 7 can be visualized spacially in the sense that a $(1 \times p)$ vector, $\mathbf{x}'$ of scores for a single individual, can be represented by a point in a p-dimensional Euclidean space, a common approach to cluster analysis is to consider the distances, or squares of distances, between such points. Problems of metrics and of possible correlation between variables arise here. The latter, if necessary, can be overcome by an orthogonal transformation of the variables (say by a principal component analysis of covariance) into a new set, which are uncorrelated but in which the distances between pairs of points remain unchanged. A component analysis would also enable one to reduce the number of original variables to a more manageable set if this were desirable. On the other hand if the original variables have different metrics and it is thought desirable to standardize them this may be accomplished by using Mahalanobis' generalized distance function, D^2 (Rao, 1952), though this does not preserve the original relative distances between the points.

One method of cluster analysis, based on the squares of distances between points, is described by Edwards and Cavalli-Sforza (1963). They use the fact 'that the variance of n points on a line is equal to the sum of all the squared distances between points taken two at a time, divided by n^2'. They proceed to divide the points into two clusters for which the 'within-clusters' sum of squares is a minimum. Each cluster obtained in this way can be further subdivided into two, and so by continued bifurcation a tree-diagram is obtained. However, use of the method is very limited by the fact that even for relatively small n the amount of sorting involved becomes prohibitively large.

The most elaborate attack on the problem of clustering, known to the author, is that by Friedman and Rubin (1966). These authors work with the well-known matrix identity

$$\mathbf{T} = \mathbf{W} + \mathbf{B}$$

where $\mathbf{T}$ is the total $p \times p$ matrix of corrected sums of squares and cross-products for n subjects on p variables and $\mathbf{W}$ and $\mathbf{B}$ are the corresponding 'within' and 'between' matrices for a given number, g, of subgroups. For some preassigned value of g the members of the composite sample are allocated to groups arbitrarily or on the basis of prior information. Then, provided that $p < n - g$, so that $\mathbf{W}^{-1}$ exists, subjects are moved one at a time from one group to another with a view to maximizing a criterion. Two criteria in particular are considered, namely

$$| \mathbf{W}^{-1}\mathbf{T} | = | \mathbf{I} + \mathbf{W}^{-1}\mathbf{B} |, \text{ and}$$
$$\text{trace } (\mathbf{W}^{-1}\mathbf{T}) = p + \text{trace } (\mathbf{W}^{-1}\mathbf{B}).$$

Of the two, the authors express some preference for the former, since it is invariant under non-singular linear transformation of the data. The arbitrariness in Friedman and Rubin's procedure lies in the choice of a value to assign to g in the first instance; but given an efficient computer program different values can be tried and the results can be assessed on prior knowledge of the variables and the acceptability of the subgroups found.

TWO EXAMPLES OF CLUSTERING PROCEDURES

It would be impossible in a short chapter to review the great variety of clustering procedures in current use, and results given by just two methods are reported here.

Method A

The principle behind this method is that of maximizing the interaction F-ratio in a profile analysis. The method begins by finding scores for each patient, in a composite sample, on the principal components for the variables or rating scales. Using these scores, interpoint distances (Euclidean space) are calculated for the patients, taken in pairs. These are examined and a number of patients (generally only 3 or 4 to begin with) who are far apart from each other, are chosen as nuclei for the formation of clusters. The other patients are then allocated to the nucleus to which they are nearest and a profile analysis is carried out on the resultant clusters. Borderline cases are then moved from one cluster to another, by considering their distances from the means of the groups, in an effort to maximize the interaction F-ratio in the analysis. A program, for the London University Atlas Computer, was written for this analysis by Mr. M. R. B. Clarke and it was tried out on a sample of 67 psychotic patients who previously had been allocated by a psychiatric colleague, Dr. J. Wing, to one or other of the four diagnostic categories:

A. Non-paranoids (patients 1–22).
B. Paranoids: with thought disorder prominent (patients 23–41).

C. Paranoids: with delusions prominent (patients 42–54).

D. Paranoids: with hallucinations prominent (patients 55–67).

The program gave results which agreed fairly well with the psychiatrist's diagnosis when five categories were assumed, the data consisting of ratings for the patients on each of nine psychiatric scales.

The five clusters (I–V) derived from the computer analysis included the following patients:

I	1	2	3	4	5	7	8	9	10	11	12	
	13	14	15	16	17	18	19	20	21	22		(A)
					(30, 62)							
II	23	24	27	29	37	40						(B)
			(49, 58)									
III	26	28	31	32	33	34	35	36	38	39	41	(B)
					(6, 51 53, 59)							
IV	55	56	57	60	61	63	64	65	66	67		(D)
					(25, 43 46 54)							
V	42	44	45	47	48	50	52					(C)

Of these, cluster I agrees closely with the clinicians' Group A, while III, IV, and V agree relatively well with Groups B, D, and C respectively. The computer has thus given a clustering near enough to that given by the clinicians to make a re-examination of the latter's diagnoses interesting, in particular the clinicians' Group B has been divided into two subgroups.

Method B

The second method to be illustrated begins with a matrix of similarity coefficients (on a 0–1 scale) between pairs of subjects. The program searches the matrix, omitting diagonal cells, for the largest coefficient, records it, and notes the two subjects concerned. It then averages the coefficients for each variable for these subjects and puts the averages in the row and column of the subject that appears first in the matrix. Simultaneously it eliminates the other subject from the matrix. When this is done a search is made for the largest coefficient of similarity in the resulting matrix and the analysis proceeds as before. For each stage of the analysis the results of the search are printed out. The experimenter then examines the print-out and constructs the clusters step by step. The great advantage of the method is that a decision need not be made in advance concerning the number of clusters. The experimenter can stop the clustering process at any stage he wishes, that is, at any given value of similarity.

This method was also applied to Dr. J. Wing's sample of 67 psychotic patients and gave the following clusters, each of which has internal similarity coefficients equal to, or greater than, the values in brackets.

LOWEST SIMILARITY COEFFICIENT					CLUSTER							DR. WING'S CLASSI-FICATION
(0·452)	1	2	3	4	5	6	8	9	12	13	16 19	(A)
						(30)						
(0·643)	7	10	11	14	15	17	18	20	21	22		(A)
					(25 35 36 41, 62)							
(0·482)	43	46	51	53	54							(C)
	56	57	61	63	64	66	(32)					(D)
(0·563)	23	27	29	40								(B)
	55	58	59	60	67	(49)						(D)
(0·822)	33	38	39									(B)
	(24, 65)											
(0·531)	45	48	50	52								(C)
(0·427)	42	44	47	(C);					26	28		(B)
(0·744)	31	34	37									(B)

This analysis separates Dr. Wing's non-paranoids (A) into two clusters the second of which contains four patients from Group B (paranoids with thought disorder). These two groups would coalesce were the similarity to be reduced to (0·331).

Among the remaining clusters Wing's Group B is widely divided; Group C somewhat less so, while his Group D is largely accounted for by just two of the clusters given by the program. To repeat, this type of clustering has the advantage that at each stage of the analysis one can see how the clustering is evolving, and at each stage one knows the degree of similarity in the clusters already formed.

In a recent review article Gower (1968) compares three clustering methods—those by Sokal and Michener (1958), Edwards and Cavalli-Sforza (1963), and Williams and Lambert (1960)—and shows that the clustering criteria of all three can be interpreted in terms of the distances between the centroids of the clusters. Of the three methods he recommends the first for general purpose classification, and it is of interest to note that this method closely resembles the second applied above to Dr. Wing's data, though Sokal and Michener's method is probably preferable as it uses weighted averages.

In conclusion, it is only fair to say that the results given by both the methods of clustering employed above are far from clear-cut. To note this is only to be realistic for, in the writer's experience, the problem of satisfactorily classifying psychiatric patients is likely to be with us for many years to come. Its solution will depend not only on the ingenuity of the statistician but also on the ability of psychiatrists to find measures which differentiate efficiently between different types of illness.

REFERENCES

ANDERSON, T. W. (1962) *Introduction to Multivariate Statistical Analysis*, New York.

BARTLETT, M. S. (1947) Multivariate analysis, *J. roy. statist. Soc.*, **9**, 176.

BARTLETT, M. S. (1965) Multivariate statistics, in *Theoretical and Mathematical Biology*, eds. Morowitz, H. J., and Waterman, T. E., New York.

BIRNBAUM, A., and MAXWELL, A. E. (1961) Classification procedures based on Bayes's formula, *Appl. Statist.*, **9**, 152.

BOX, G. E. P. (1949) A general distribution theory for a class of likelihood criteria, *Biometrika*, **36**, 317.

BOX, G. E. P. (1954) Some theorems on quadratic forms applied in the study of analysis of variance problems: I. Effect of inequality of variance in the one-way classification, *Ann. math. Statist.*, **25**, 290.

BOX, G. E. P. (1954) Some theorems on quadratic forms applied in the study of analysis of variance problems: II. Effects of inequality of variance and of correlation between errors in the two-way classification, *Ann. math. Statist.*, **25**, 484.

EDWARDS, A. W. F., and CAVALLI-SFORZA, L. L. (1963) A method for cluster analysis, *Biometrics*, **21**, 362.

FISHER, R. A. (1936) The use of multiple measurements in taxonomic problems, *Ann. Eugen. (Lond.)*, **7**, 179.

FRIEDMAN, H. P., and RUBIN, J. (1966) *On Some Invariant Criteria for Grouping Data*, I.B.M. New York Scientific Centre, Technical Report.

GEISSER, S. (1964) Posterior odds for multivariate normal classifications, *J. roy. statist. Soc.*, **26**, 69.

GOWER, J. C. (1968) A comparison of some methods of cluster analysis, *Biometrics*, **23**, 62.

GREENHOUSE, S. W., and GEISSER, S. (1959) On methods in the analysis of profile data, *Psychometrica*, **24**, 95.

HEALY, M. J. R. (1965) Descriptive uses of discriminant functions, in *Mathematics and Computer Science in Biology and Medicine*, London, H.M.S.O.

HECK, D. L. (1960) Charts of some upper percentage points in the distribution of the large characteristic root, *Ann. math. Statist.*, **31**, 625.

HILLS, M. (1966) Allocation rules and their error rates, *J. roy. statist. Soc.*, **28**, 1.

JOYCE, T., and CHANNON, C. (1966) Classifying market survey respondents, *Appl. Statist.*, **15**, 191.

LAWLEY, D. N., and MAXWELL, A. E. (1963) *Factor Analysis as a Statistical Method*, London.

MACNAUGHTON-SMITH, P. (1965) *Some Statistical and Other Numerical Techniques for Classifying Individuals*, Home Office Research Unit, London, H.M.S.O.

MAHALANOBIS, P. C. (1936) On the generalised distance in statistics, *Proc. Nat. Inst. Soc. India*, **12**, 49.

MAXWELL, A. E. (1961) Canonical variate analysis when the variables are dichotomous, *Educational and Psychol. Measurement*, **21**, 259.

MORRISON, D. F. (1967) *Multivariate Statistical Methods*, New York.

RAO, C. R. (1948) Utilisation of multiple measurements in problems of biological classifications, *J. roy. statist. Soc.*, **10**, 159.

RAO, C. R. (1952) *Advanced Statistical Methods in Biometric Research*, New York.

RAO, C. R., and SLATER, P. (1949) Multivariate analysis applied to differences between neurotic groups, *Brit. J. statist. Psychol.* **2**, 17.

SLATER, P. (1960) Canonical analysis of discriminance, in *Experiments in Personality*, Vol. 2, ed. Eysenck, H. J., London.

M

SNEATH, P. H. A., and SOKAL, R. R. (1963) *Principles of Numerical Taxonomy*, London.

SOKAL, R. R., and MICHENER, C. D. (1958) A statistical method for evaluating systematic relationships, *Univ. Kansas Sci. Bull.*, **38**, 1409.

WILLIAMS, W. T., and LAMBERT, J. M. (1959) Multivariate methods in plant ecology. I. Association analysis in plant communities, *J. Ecol.*, **47**, 83.

WILLIAMS, W. T., and LAMBERT, J. M. (1960) Multivariate methods in plant ecology. II. The use of an electronic digital computer for association analysis, *J. Ecol.*, **48**, 689.

WISHART, J. (1955) Multivariate analysis, *Appl. Statist.*, **4**, 51.

13

MODELS OF SURVIVORSHIP

D. KODLIN

INTRODUCTION

MODELS of human survival are essentially descriptive devices. While they are useful in providing summary statements derived from an incomplete set of observations, they shed little light on biological mechanisms leading to death. Nevertheless, as tools of 'data reduction' they play a useful role in epidemiology and in clinical problems of treatment evaluation. The latter area of application has become more prominent throughout the years, and this fact is reflected by a preponderance of statistical tools specially geared to follow-up of patients under heavy risk.

From the basic notion that survival time is a quantitative variable, it follows naturally that one would attempt to find simple frequency distributions of survival times, so that the parameter(s) of the distribution that appears to fit a given set of observations can be used as a concise summary of these observations. The procedure is thus quite similar to the familiar methods of estimating the mean and variance as parameters of the normal distribution when dealing with such quantitative variables as height, weight, or blood pressure.

A typical complication arises from the fact that there is truncation, that is, survival of some persons to the end of the follow-up period; if 'intake' is staggered over the follow-up period the truncation time will vary from person to person. A straightforward computation of the mean survival time is therefore not possible. However, the quantity can still be estimated by first obtaining estimates of the parameters of the distribution (which is possible in the presence of truncation), and then computing the mean, a known function of the parameters.

In this chapter, we will explore this notion with the aid of a few examples of epidemiological concern. Much elaboration can be found in the related area of industrial 'life testing', easily accessible from the bibliography of Mendenhall (1958) and the monograph by Barlow and Proschan (1965).

It is to be hoped that the examples will also suffice to indicate, at least roughly, the conditions under which the 'non-parametric' approaches to survival are preferable. These begin with the classical life table technique, still the subject of theoretical study (Chiang, 1961) and, when two groups being followed for survival are compared, involve ranking procedures such as the Dixon–Mood sign test (Armitage, 1959), a generalized Wilcoxon test developed by Gehan (1965) and the Kolmogorov–Smirnov test recently explored by Mantel (1968). An interesting version of the actuarial (life table) technique is Kaplan and Meier's *product-limit* estimate (1958). Quite generally, non-parametric tests are less efficient than parametric ones, and Armitage (1959) finds this to be true when comparing the sign test and the Kaplan–Meier estimator with the parametric procedure assuming the true distribution of survival times to be the exponential distribution. The latter, often admittedly chosen for mathematical convenience, enters even into versions of the life table technique when one deals with the problem of truncation (withdrawal) and 'competing risk' (Chiang, 1961; Neyman, 1950). Of greater importance is the fact that the distribution is quite satisfactory in certain applications of interest (*vide infra*) and can be easily extended. It thus provides a convenient starting point for our discussion.

GENERAL DESCRIPTION OF TWO SIMPLE LAWS OF SURVIVAL

The most elementary survival time distributions (in the mathematical sense) are the exponential and its extension, the 'linear-exponential' distribution. They are perhaps also the most useful in our context. The former, recurring in many engineering applications, is treated in detail in most statistical texts covering this field, the latter is a relative newcomer; brief discussions have been given by Broadbent (1958) and Flehinger and Lewis (1959), while the writer has treated the subject in greater detail (Kodlin, 1967).

The Exponential Distribution

If a population dies off with a constant annual mortality so that for each time interval $(t, t + 1)$ the mortality rate is

$$m(t, t + 1) = 1 - e^{-c}, \qquad (1)$$

where c is a constant and e the base of the natural logarithm, then one can show that the underlying survival time distribution is

$$f(t) = ce^{-ct}, \qquad (2)$$

and the fraction surviving to time t is

$$s(t) = e^{-ct}. \qquad (3)$$

This is the familiar 'law of exponential decay' and one would perhaps suspect that it would only describe such elementary processes as the decay of radioactive atoms or that of virus particles. Before demonstrating that the law may hold for human populations also, at least over a considerable span of follow-up time, a few technical remarks may be useful:

1. A plot of the functions (1), (2), and (3) against time t, for various values of c, is most useful. They can be easily worked out with the aid of a table of e^{-x} found in most table collections and on some specialized pocket slide rules such as Aristo No. 868. Advice to plot applies to observational material as well; this is of particular convenience in the scanning of large bodies of data such as international compilations of 'end results' in cancer therapy. The *1963 International Symposium* on this topic contains not only illustrative material but also a concise account, by the editor S. J. Cutler, of simple life table computations that may be used to obtain, from one's own data, *observed* fractions surviving to t which, when plotted against t, can be compared with function (3).

2. As long as the parameter c in formula (1) remains less than about 0·1, a good approximation for $1 - e^{-c}$ is c, so that

$$m(t, t + 1) \simeq c. \tag{4}$$

That is to say, the meaning of the parameter c is simply the constant annual mortality.

3. If, in formula (2), we take the natural logarithm on both sides we obtain

$$- \ln s(t) = ct. \tag{5}$$

Thus, the negative logarithm of the observed fraction surviving to t, when plotted against follow-up time t, will give a straight line, if, and only if, the law holds.

4. The familiar 'person-year rate' is an estimator of c, in fact a maximum likelihood estimate (Littell, 1952). As Sheps (1966) has pointed out repeatedly, the use of this estimator should be restricted to follow-up data showing evidence of a *constant* annual rate of response. We shall demonstrate the poor performance of this estimator when this condition does not hold.

The 'Linear-Exponential' Distribution

In contrast to the exponential distribution (which might, more appropriately in this context, be called the *constant exponential*, being made up of a *constant* term c and an *exponential* term e^{-ct} (see formula (2)) a more complex distribution of survival times is obtained if the annual mortality $m(t, t + 1)$ increases in time according to the formula

$$m(t, t + 1) = 1 - e^{- (c + \frac{1}{2}k + kt)}.$$

As long as the exponent $c + \frac{1}{2}k + kt$ remains less than 0·1, this can be written as

$$m(t, t + 1) \simeq c + \tfrac{1}{2}k + kt. \tag{6}$$

We thus have, in contrast to (4), a linear rise in annual mortality with 'initial' mortality (year zero to one) of $c + \frac{1}{2}k$ and slope k.

The meaning of the two parameters is thus easy to remember:

1. $c + \frac{1}{2}k$ is the initial mortality rate in the first year of follow-up.
2. k is the 'annual increment in annual mortality'.

Furthermore, if k goes to zero, (6) goes to (4) and the two distributions become identical. This can also be seen from the expression for the distribution of survival times, namely

$$f(t) = (c + kt)e^{-(ct + \frac{1}{2}kt^2)}, \tag{7}$$

which reduces to (2) if k goes to zero. The distribution is 'linear-exponential' in the sense that it is composed of a linear term $c + kt$ and an exponential one, $e^{-(ct + \frac{1}{2}kt^2)}$.

Corresponding to (3), the fraction surviving to t is

$$s(t) = e^{-(ct + \frac{1}{2}kt^2)}, \tag{8}$$

and corresponding to (5)

$$-\frac{\ln s(t)}{t} = c + \frac{1}{2}kt. \tag{9}$$

Thus, the negative logarithm of the observed fraction surviving to t, dividing by t, will, when plotted against t, give a straight line with slope $\frac{1}{2}k$. Note that, as k goes to zero, formula (9) goes to c, a result also obtained from (5) if both sides of (5) are divided by t.

In conjunction with FIGURE 15, the foregoing remarks may suffice as background for the following section. The reader may find technical details such as the estimation of parameters c and k and their standard errors in the references quoted. Unless the data are scanty, fairly good estimates of c and k can be obtained from plots of (6) or (9). Such graphical orientation provides a useful check on computational estimates, and when differences between population groups are large, the graphical estimates may be quite sufficient in summarizing the survival pattern of each group.

APPLICATIONS

In FIGURE 16 data from the Metropolitan Life Insurance Company (Robb and Marks, 1953) are plotted on a logarithmic scale. Evidently, the straight line relation postulated by formula (5) does hold and one may thus conclude that persons, after diagnosis of 'arteriosclerotic and hypertensive heart disease' is made, experience survival times according to the simple law of exponential decay. In particular, as the c-values of 0·069 and 0·072 indicate, the annual, constant, mortality rate is 6·9 per cent for the uncomplicated cases and the label 'coronary occlusion' raises the rate only slightly to 7·2 per cent. In contrast, 'renal or cerebral involvement' raises the rate to 18 per cent. For significance tests see Armitage (1959).

One may speculate as to the reason for this phenomenon. If the vascular system contains a number of 'critical spots' functional impairment of which leads to death, and if the probability of 'hitting' such a 'target' (by embolism producing obstruction or by mechanical forces resulting in rupture, perhaps) is constant in time, one would expect in fact 'one-hit kinetics', that is to say, exponential survival (Timofeeff-Ressovsky and Zimmer, 1947).

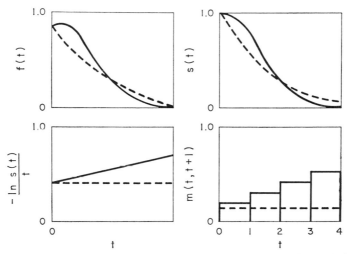

FIG. 15. General shape of the exponential distribution (broken line), of the linear-exponential distribution (solid line) and of functions derived from them.

$f(t)$ = frequency distribution of survival time t.
$s(t)$ = fraction surviving to t.
$m(t, t + 1)$ = annual mortality rate between t and $t + 1$.

Irrespective of the merits of such interpretation, the fact remains that the exponential distribution appears to be a useful descriptive device of survival of persons suffering from a disease that is one of the leading causes of death.

The simple exponential distribution is by no means enough to account for survival patterns observed after diagnosis (and treatment) of conditions that produce annual mortality rates in excess of 20 per cent, such as sarcomas and other malignancies. Here the patients are likely to be heterogeneous ('cured–uncured') and, in addition, the pooling of cases with different initial stages of severity will complicate the pattern from the start. Models attempting to account for some of these effects (Boag, 1949; Berkson and Gage, 1952; Sampford, 1954; Kodlin, 1961; Cutler and Axtell, 1963) will not be discussed further here, since they are of more interest to clinical research than to epidemiology. The paper of Zelen (1966) should be mentioned, however, as an example of model building that incorporates at least some biological elements such as cell growth and destruction as determinants of survival in leukaemia.

In general, marked systematic deviations from postulated simple distributions such as the exponential, log normal or linear exponential (the latter to

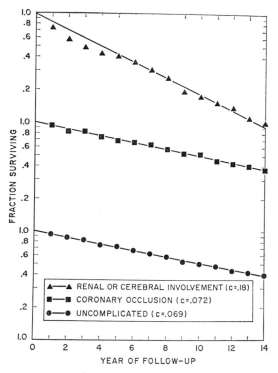

FIG. 16. Observed fraction surviving, 'after diagnosis of arteriosclerotic and hypertensive heart disease'; data from the Metropolitan Life Insurance Company. Solid lines: expected fraction surviving under exponential model (constant annual mortality c). Logarithmic plot according to formula (5) of text.

be discussed in more detail below) may lead one to rely on one of the non-parametric approaches listed in the introduction. Some investigators seem to feel that this recourse is advisable also in case of scanty information where the systematic nature of deviations is hard to establish. Unfortunately, the loss in efficiency hurts most in such cases.

Most populations of interest to epidemiology are, of course, subject to risks much smaller than those we have discussed so far. Of particular relevance in this respect is the follow-up information from Hiroshima and Nagasaki (Beebe, Ishida, and Jablon, 1962; Jablon, Ishida, and Beebe, 1964; Jablon, Ishida, and Yamasaki, 1965), since it is concerned with a population of about

100,000 persons followed now for more than 15 years. On such numbers one would have the opportunity to observe the occurrence of systematic deviations from postulated laws of survival and if such deviations do not occur or are of a minor nature one would strongly expect such laws to be of more general use in the description of population survival. FIGURE 17 shows the observed and expected survival for a few subgroups of unexposed persons, covering the period 1950–64. The agreement between observation and expectation from the linear-exponential model is excellent. In contrast, the 'con-

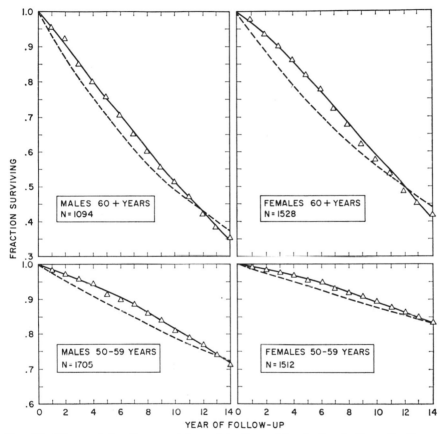

FIG. 17. Observed fraction surviving; data from Atomic Bomb Casualty Commission, updated to 1964. Oldest age groups, 'not in city' (unexposed). N = initial size of sample. Solid line: expected fraction surviving under linear-exponential model (linear increase in annual mortality). Broken line: expected fraction surviving under exponential model (constant annual mortality).

stant exponential' (broken line), with parameter c estimated by the 'person-year' rate, shows considerable deviations, and provides a description of the data only in the sense that it replaces the linearly increasing mortality rate by a constant rate. In the process of doing so the 'initial' mortality rate is overestimated and the 'late' mortality rate is underestimated.

Parameter estimates for c and k for the curves of FIGURE 17 are of the order of $c = 0.01$, $k = 0.001$ for the age group 50–59 years and $c = 0.04$, $k = 0.004$ for the age group 60+ years. According to formula (6), the initial mortality is therefore

$$m(0,1) = c + \tfrac{1}{2}k = 0.0105$$

for the first age group, and

$$m(0,1) = c + \tfrac{1}{2}k = 0.0420$$

for the second one.

In other words, 1–4 per cent die in the first year of follow-up. Similarly, the mortality between year 10 and 11 would be

$$m(10,11) = c + \tfrac{1}{2}k + 10k,$$

that is, 0.0205 and 0.0820, respectively.

FIGURE 18 demonstrates the fact that differences between exposure groups are reflected by differences in the parameters which can therefore be used for

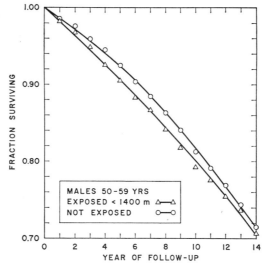

FIG. 18. Observed and expected fraction surviving; data source as in FIGURE 17. Contrast between two exposure groups, aged 50–59. Solid lines: expected fraction surviving under linear-exponential model (linear increase in annual mortality).

comparison between the groups. FIGURES 19 and 20 show that, as one moves to younger age groups, the parameter k goes to zero so that the 'constant exponential' holds, and comparisons between groups can be made by the parameter c (constant annual mortality), now properly estimated by the

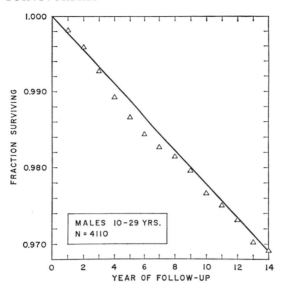

FIG. 19. Observed and expected fraction surviving; data source as in FIGURE 17. Younger age group, 'not in city' (unexposed). Satisfactory expectations from exponential model (solid line).

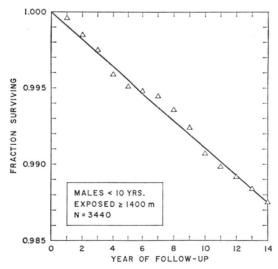

FIG. 20. Observed and expected fraction surviving; data source as in FIGURE 17. Younger age group, exposed. Satisfactory expectations from exponential model (solid line).

person-year rate. The purpose of presenting some of these data in our context is simply to point out that this material (representing perhaps the most extensive effort of follow-up ever undertaken) seems to be subject to rather straightforward description.

The satisfactory performance of our two distributions on a Japanese population group leaves us with the question whether they may perform equally well on other groups. Unfortunately, relevant material is hard to find. Routine record keeping on 'cohorts' in the context of large-scale insurance schemes is not likely to be of the quality that can be obtained in *ad hoc* efforts such as those made in Japan. However, one may perhaps argue that gross effects such as the high risk of chromate workers (Taylor, 1966), for instance, could be assessed when their survival is evaluated in comparison with that of the general working population, *all information* coming from the same source such as the Old Age and Survivors Insurance of the United States.

Data from this source (Ciocco, Mancuso, and Thompson, 1965) have been plotted in FIGURE 21. While the two youngest age groups follow a linear-exponential distribution, the two older ones show a sudden deviation at year 12, most likely an artifact, to judge from its precipitous and simultaneous appearance. Indeed, the material has so far been published only for a four-

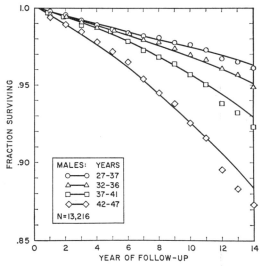

FIG. 21. Observed fractions surviving; data from Old Age and Survivors Insurance, various age groups. Solid lines: expectations from linear-exponential model (linear increase in annual mortality).

year span, perhaps an indication that the authors have been discouraged by sufficient similar inconsistencies. Nevertheless, a plot of Taylor's data (1966) for comparable age groups, which is not reproduced on FIGURE 21, would show a convincing separation of the chromate workers whose excess risk Taylor had previously established in relation to vital statistics rates only.

While the example may, perhaps, still demonstrate the creditable performance of the analytical tools under consideration, it is most useful in drawing attention to the fact that unique opportunities for risk evaluation in the area of industrial medicine are lost when such evaluation appears as an afterthought, rather than as a carefully nursed objective of social institutions.

In conclusion, some general remarks are perhaps in order, once more, concerning the purpose of survivorship models. When we say that they are descriptive devices we have in mind that the descriptive summary will be used as a means for comparison between groups of persons, *on the basis of evidence from the follow-up period*. More sophisticated models are different in this respect since their merit will be judged *by their ability to make non-trivial predictions as to the future (unobserved) state of affairs*. Clearly, the statement that 'cases of coronary occlusion have a 7 per cent annual mortality for each of the fourteen follow-up years' implies nothing as to the future course of events. Similarly, the finding that an age group of persons under 10 years dies off over the follow-up period of fourteen years at a constant annual mortality rate of $c = 0.003$ does not imply that this rate will hold when the group has reached an advanced age. Indeed, the mean survival time for a group subject to such a rate continuously would be $1/c = 333$ years, an unreasonable expectation of life.

However, if the ultimate purpose of survival time analysis is to assist in the identification of life-shortening hazards and in decision making for their control while knowledge is incomplete, then only the 'lesson of the past' is relevant and the sooner and the more succinctly it can be stated the more useful it would appear to be. Beyond that, Broadbent's observation (1958) that milk bottles break down according to the linear-exponential law, and the present contention that older persons follow such a pattern over more than a decade should remind us that from the use of such models a deep insight into the mechanics of failure is not to be expected.

REFERENCES

ARMITAGE, P. (1959) The comparison of survival curves, *J. roy. statist. Soc.*, Ser. A., **122**, 279.

BARLOW, R. E., and PROSCHAN, F. (1965) *Mathematical Theory of Reliability*, New York.

BEEBE, G. W., ISHIDA, M., and JABLON, S. (1962) Studies of the mortality of A-bomb survivors. 1. Plan of study and mortality in the medical subsample (Selection I), 1950–1958, *Radiation Research*, **16**, 253.

BERKSON, J., and GAGE, R. P. (1952) Survival curve for cancer patients following treatment, *J. Amer. statist. Ass.*, **47**, 501.

BOAG, J. W. (1949) Maximum likelihood estimates of the proportion of patients cured by cancer therapy, *J. roy. statist. Soc.*, Ser. B., **11**, 15.

180　　　　　　　　　　　　　　　　　　　　　　　　　　　　　　　ANALYSIS

BROADBENT, S. (1958) Simple mortality rates, *J. roy. statist. Soc.*, Ser. C., **7**, 86.
CHIANG, C. L. (1961) A stochastic study of the life table and its applications. III. The follow-up study with the consideration of competing risk, *Biometrics*, **17**, 57.
CIOCCO, A., MANCUSO, T., and THOMPSON, D. J. (1965) Four years' mortality experience of a segment of the United States working population, *Amer. J. publ. Hlth*, **55**, 587.
CUTLER, S. J., and AXTELL, L. M. (1963) Partitioning of a patient population with respect to different mortality risks, *J. Amer. statist. Ass.*, **58**, 701.
FLEHINGER, B. J., and LEWIS, P. A. (1959) Two-parameter lifetime distributions for reliability studies of renewal processes, *I.B.M. J. of Research and Development*, **3**, 58.
GEHAN, E. A. (1965) A generalised Wilcoxon test for comparing arbitrarily single-censored samples, *Biometrika*, **52**, 203.
INTERNATIONAL SYMPOSIUM ON END RESULTS IN CANCER THERAPY (1964) ed. CUTLER, S. J., *Nat. Cancer Inst. Monogr.*, **15**, Washington, D.C.
JABLON, S., ISHIDA, M., and BEEBE, G. W. (1964) Studies of the mortality of A-bomb survivors. 2. Mortality in Selections I and II, 1950–1959, *Radiation Research*, **21**, 423.
JABLON, S., ISHIDA, M., and YAMASAKI, M. (1965) Studies of the mortality of A-bomb survivors. 3. Description of the sample and mortality, 1950–1960, *Radiation Research*, **25**, 25.
KAPLAN, E. L., and MEIER, P. (1958) Nonparametric estimation from incomplete observations, *J. Amer. statist. Ass.*, **53**, 457.
KODLIN, D. (1961) Survival time analysis for treatment evaluation in cancer therapy, *Cancer Res.*, **21**, 1103.
KODLIN, D. (1967) A new response time distribution, *Biometrics*, **23**, 227.
LITTELL, A. S. (1952) Estimation of the T-year survival rate from follow-up studies over a limited period of time, *Hum. Biol.*, **24**, 87.
MANTEL, N. (1968) Kolmogorov–Smirnov tests and Réyni's modification, *Biometrics*, **24**, 1018.
MENDENHALL, W. (1958) A bibliography of life testing and related topics, *Biometrika*, **45**, 521.
NEYMAN, J. (1950) *First Course in Probability and Statistics*, New York.
ROBB, G. P., and MARKS, H. H. (1953) What happens to men disabled by heart disease, *Trans. Ass. Life Insur. med. Dir. Amer.*, **37**, 171.
SAMPFORD, M. R. (1954) The estimation of response-time distributions. III.Truncation and survival, *Biometrics*, **10**, 531.
SHEPS, M. C. (1966) Characteristics of a ratio used to estimate failure rates: occurrences per person—year of exposure, *Biometrics*, **22**, 310.
SHEPS, M. C. (1966) On the person years concept in epidemiology and demography, *Milbank mem. Fd Quart.*, **44**, 69.
TAYLOR, F. (1966) The relationship of mortality and duration of employment as reflected by a cohort of chromate workers, *Amer. J. publ. Hlth*, **56**, 218.
TIMOFEEFF-RESSOVSKY, N. W., and ZIMMER, K. G. (1947) Das Trefferprinzip in der Biologie, in *Biophysik*, Vol. 1, Hirzel, S., Leipzig.
ZELEN, M. (1966) Application of exponential models to problems in cancer research, *J. roy. statist. Soc.*, Ser. A., **129**, 368.

14

MODELS IN HEALTH SERVICES PLANNING

Vicente Navarro and Roger D. Parker

INTRODUCTION

THIS chapter presents some of the mathematical analytical models used either in operations research or systems analysis that have been used in health services planning. Emphasis is placed on the description of Markov models—a Markovian planning model is described as a tool for predicting requirements for resources, for calculating changes in those resources in simulated situations, and for estimating the optimum alternative for the constraint chosen to reach a specified goal. A practical example describing the planning of personal health services for patients with cardiovascular diseases illustrates the three applications of the model.

A *system* is defined as a 'regularly interacting or interdependent group of items forming a unified whole', and 'a group of interacting bodies under the influence of related forces . . .'[1] A system of personal health services consists of interdependent elements, such as physicians, nurses, facilities, and other resources, that interact under the influence of diverse forces with the community they serve.

Furthermore, the elements of any health system can be grouped in subsystems that depend on the criteria for the grouping—for example, first contact or primary medical care, specialist or consultant medical care, community hospital care, teaching hospital care, etc. The term *subsystem* is interchangeable with the term *level* or *state of care*.

The state of a health services system can be defined by the values of those variables that describe its elements—for example, the prevalence of a particular disease or the number of available hospital beds, as well as by the process of transformation in the system whereby inputs are translated into outputs.

The *input* into each state can be measured by the number of entries, that is, persons or conditions, as determined by the actual 'demand' for services per unit of time. For example, a patient who twice visits a consultant specialist during one year because of otitis media constitutes an entry to the consultant care state, with two visits for entry into that state during the year. If need is

---

[1] WEBSTER, N. (1967) *Seventh New Collegiate Dictionary*.

preferred to actual demand, the input in the model can be changed to a desired potential demand.

As Last (1963) explains, such a shift assumes that need—the submerged part of the iceberg of disease—can be translated into demand. The conceptual distinction between those two approaches has been discussed elsewhere (Navarro, 1970). The parameters that define this input will depend on the criterion chosen to define such measures of ill health as disease, disability, dissatisfaction, and discomfort (White, 1967).

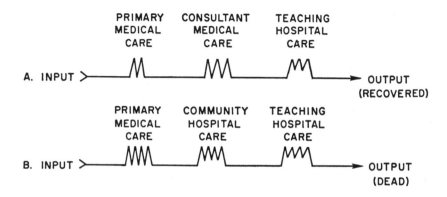

UTILIZATION STRATEGIES

A. 2 visits per entry to Primary Medical Care
    3 visits per entry to Consultant Medical Care
    3 days per entry to Teaching Hospital Care

B. 4 visits per entry to Primary Medical Care
    4 days per entry to Community Hospital Care
    4 days per entry to Teaching Hospital Care

FIG. 22. Utilization strategies.

The *output* of each state can be measured by the number of discharges or outcomes from each unit of time. Alternative outcomes might include: dead/alive, diseased/healthy, disabled/fit, dissatisfied/satisfied, or uncomfortable/comfortable.

The *throughput* system represents the time movement of patients through the several states of the system. This movement within the system can be made between two units within the same state of care (a transfer) or between units of different states (a referral).

Transfers and referrals document the movement or flow of people within a health services system and the dynamic relationships among its different states and units. The series of referrals and transfers experienced by each patient defines the utilization strategy employed (Reinke, 1970). Thus, the throughput of the entire system can be defined as the totality of utilization for all patients. FIGURE 22 shows two examples of utilization strategies.

MODELS BASED ON THE KNOWLEDGE OF THE PERFORMANCE OF THE SYSTEM

Planning personal health services can be based upon analysis of the performance or the structure of the system. In the methods based upon its performance, the resources required are determined by the amount and type needed to achieve a certain output, called product output, which is measured in terms of performance, such as reduction or control of death, disease, disability, discomfort, etc. In those methods based on the structure of the system, the output is defined as process output and measured in terms of services provided or population covered. The relationship between input and output in the system performance method is called 'effectiveness';[2] the same relationship between input and output in the system structure method is called 'efficiency'.

Unfortunately, little is known about the effectiveness of different health services. Most analytical studies of these have been concerned with productivity, expressed in terms of efficiency, but not with effectiveness. The paucity of effectiveness studies is due to present limitations in the knowledge of the relationships between the different variables involved in the output as well as in the input of the system. In most cases the relationships between the system and the performance are not known; even less is known about the methods of quantifying these. There is no evidence, for example, that in providing X units of prenatal care one will save Y children's lives. It is in the study of these relationships that epidemiological studies are greatly needed. Only in those cases with a known quantifiable relationship between input and product output, such as kidney dialysis and prevention of death in certain cases of renal failure, is it possible to use techniques, such as cost-benefit or cost-effectiveness analysis, that require this knowledge (Klarman, Francis, and Rosenthal, 1968). Otherwise, the usefulness of the technique is conditional on the validity of the assumptions of this relationship.

The absence of objective standards to measure the relationships between systems and their product output explains the use of subjective measures such as the opinion of experts. The *Centro de Estudios de Desarrollo* (C.E.N.D.E.S.), the Pan American Health Organization (Ahumada *et al.*, 1965) and the United States Public Health Service (Division of Indian Health, 1966) have defined planning methods that require these experts' judgement about the vulnerability of the disease to certain curative and preventive activities.

---

[2] Some authors prefer the term 'efficaciousness' to that of 'effectiveness'. It seems, however, that while the first term has most meaning on an individual or personal basis, the latter has a better applicability on a community basis.

N

MODELS BASED ON THE KNOWLEDGE OF THE STRUCTURE OF
THE SYSTEM: MARKOVIAN MODELS

In methods based upon the knowledge of the structure of the system it is convenient to use probabilistic models. These allow more flexibility to planners in facing a continuously changing and uncertain environment. Indeed, biological and social models are usually probabilistic in nature.[3]

With the work of Markov (1856–1922) an important step in the development of probability theory was taken. He studied a sequence of events, with a given distribution of initial probabilities, with the simple property that the probability of the next event in the sequence of trials depends only on the present outcome rather than on the outcome of previous trials (Harary and Lipstein, 1962). These situations, now called 'Markov chains', have been broadly studied, and modern expositions of Markov chains are contained in the books of Doob (1962), Feller (1957), Kemeny and Snell (1960), and Bartholomew (1967).

Since the first application of Markov chains in statistical mechanics, there have been many more applications in surprisingly diverse areas. These include the work on learning theory independently developed by Estes (1950), and Bush and Mosteller (1955); the study of changes in attitudes by Anderson (1954); the analysis of social mobility by Prais (1955) and labour mobility by Blumen, Kogan, and McCarthy (1955). In epidemiology, Marshall and Goldhammer (1955) have used Markov chains for the study of epidemiology of mental disease, and Fix and Neyman (1951) and Zahl (1955) have used it for the study of survival after treatment of cancer. In planning personal health services, Navarro and Parker (1968), Singer (1961), and Hope and Skrimshire (1968) have advocated the use of the Markovian chain as a mathematical model to estimate manpower and facility requirements.

A Markovian Planning Model

This model embodies a Markov chain, in which the health services states are postulated and the probabilities of going from one state to another, defined by the transitional probability matrix, determine the distribution of the number of people in the various states through time. In other words, the transitional probability of going from one health services state to another depends only on the current state that the patient is in, rather than on any previous states that have led to his current state. In addition, the transitional probabilities are assumed not to vary with time.[4]

In the present application the assumption is made that every person in the population of a defined geographical region is characterized as belonging to

[3] For a complete discussion of stochastic models, as well as a detailed survey of the whole subject of operations research and system engineering, see Flagle et al. (1960). For an analysis of their scope in medicine and biology, see Bailey (1967).

[4] For a full mathematical development of this model see Navarro (1968). For a more brief description see Navarro (1969).

one, and only one, of several mutually exclusive states of a health services system at any point in time.

The health services states shown in FIGURE 23 have been chosen arbitrarily. The state described as 'population not utilizing medical or hospital care' includes all persons who are in no other state. Moreover, it includes healthy as well as sick persons who are not under medical care in any of the other

STATES AND FLOWS

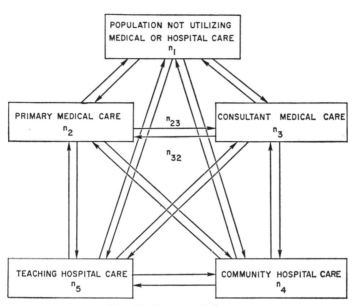

FIG. 23. States and flows.

states. Primary medical care, consultant medical care, community hospital and teaching hospital care states contain people receiving these levels of attention respectively. The number of states could be extended by adding others, as well as different units within each state. The size of the model can be extended in accord with the complexity and comprehensiveness desired, and with the availability of usable information. The population to be examined can be defined by demographic and/or epidemiological criteria.[5]

In FIGURE 23 to say that n_2 equals 20 persons means that at this moment, say $t = 0$, there are 20 persons under primary medical care.

The fractions of the population at each state, at different time periods, $P_i(t)$, equals the number of people in that health service state at that time,

[5] The choice of states in this example is arbitrary. Another choice could for example have been 'able', 'disabled', and 'dead', as in Sverdrup (1965), mentioned in Bartholomew (1967), p. 73.

$n_i(t)$, divided by the total number of people in the region served by the system at that time, $N(t)$.

For a stationary Markovian chain analysis, the transitional probabilities of going from one state to another during the fundamental time period must be calculated. The transitional probability, P_{ij}, is estimated by the number of people, n_{ij}, who are transferred from state i to state j during the defined time period, divided by the number of people n_i, in state i at the beginning of that period.

This transitional probability denotes the probability that a person who is in state i at the beginning of the defined time period will go to state j during that period. For example, if n_4, the number of people under community hospital care at a beginning point in time, is 200, and if n_{45}, the number of referrals from community hospital care to teaching hospital care measured in the week that follows, is 50, then $P_{45} = \dfrac{50}{200} = 0\cdot25$ is the estimated transitional probability per week of patients going from community hospital to teaching hospital. P_{ij} defines the movement of people within the system and reflects functional relationship among the states.

TABLE 11 presents the transitional probabilities in the described model. Each probability represents a flow between two different health services states. P_{24}, for instance, represents the probability that a person is in the primary medical care state at the beginning of the chosen time period and goes to the state of community hospital care during that time.

In this model P_{ij} is taken as known. It is determined from information about referrals within the system, [see APPENDIX 1]. It would be possible, however, for those populations where such data are available, to use P_{ij} as

TABLE 11

TRANSITIONAL PROBABILITIES

i STATE / j STATE		STATE OF MEDICAL AND HOSPITAL CARE				
STATE OF MEDICAL AND HOSPITAL CARE		Population not utilizing medical or hospital care	Primary medical care	Consultant medical care	Community hospital care	Teaching hospital care
		1	2	3	4	5
Population not utilizing medical or hospital care	1	P_{11}	P_{12}	P_{13}	P_{14}	P_{15}
Primary medical care	2	P_{21}	P_{22}	P_{23}	P_{24}	P_{25}
Consultant medical care	3	P_{31}	P_{32}	P_{33}	P_{34}	P_{35}
Community hospital care	4	P_{41}	P_{42}	P_{43}	P_{44}	P_{45}
Teaching hospital care	5	P_{51}	P_{52}	P_{53}	P_{54}	P_{55}

the dependent variable in a multiple regression analysis, considering as independent those variables which condition utilization from the standpoint of the persons, of the system, and of enabling factors.

If the fractions of the population in different health services states are known, and if the parameters that define productivity are known, the manpower and facilities required can be calculated [see APPENDIX 2].

APPLICATIONS OF THE MODEL

Prediction

Prediction is the ordinary statistical problem of forecasting. At the simplest level it involves extrapolation of past experiences into the future.

In the Markovian model, when the transitional probabilities are known, prediction is possible when only the initial fractions of the population in each state are known [see APPENDIX 3]. Prediction involves calculating the fractions of the population expected to be in the several health services states at different time periods in the future. The inputs for this model of prediction are the known current fractions in each state, and the transitional probability matrix that reflects the dynamics of the system. The outputs of the model are the estimated fractions of the population in each state at different time periods in the future. If the productivity of current resources is known it is possible to estimate the manpower and facilities required in each state in the future.

Simulation

Simulation involves observation of changes in the health services system and the repercussions of those changes on present and future utilization and resources.[6] The inputs of the model applied to simulation are the fractions of the population currently in each state and the new set of transitional probabilities that reflects simulated changes in the system. The outputs are the new patterns of utilization determined by the changes. Since the productivity of the resources is known, these new fractions in each state can be translated into a new set of resources.

Goal-seeking

Goal-seeking involves determining that alternative which minimizes 'costs' or 'changes' in resources, required to achieve, in a given time period, specified utilization patterns or specified needs for resources.

[6] The term 'simulation' used in this application is different from the similar term used in operations research, which refers to a statistical sampling method. The application of the term here is a parametric study in which, by varying the relevant transitional probabilities parametrically, one may simulate the effect of changing the patterns of referral among two or more states. The method of calculating the fractions of the population at different time periods is the same as that used in prediction [see APPENDIX 3].

The inputs of the Markovian model in goal-seeking are: the present fractions of the population in each state, the desired steady state fraction in each state for the future (or the desired number of resources in a particular state), and the selected constraint, for example, a cost constraint, a resource constraint, etc., that the alternative specified must meet. The problem is to choose that alternative, defined by a transitional probability matrix, which will minimize the constraint selected [see APPENDIX 3]. Actually there will be

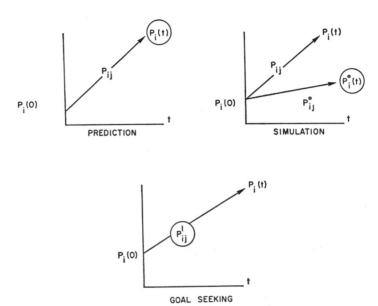

FIG. 24. Graphical representation of prediction, simulation, and goal-seeking.

an infinite number of possible alternatives in going from the present level of utilization to one desired in the future, but only one alternative will minimize the constraint selected. For instance, if the constraint is 'cost', then the alternative chosen will be the one that minimizes the cost of going from the present to the desired future level of utilization. Another example of constraint might be 'minimizing changes' and, in that case, the alternative chosen would be the one which would require minimal additional resources for each health services state at different time periods in the future.

FIGURE 24 illustrates the three applications of the Markovian model.

THE MARKOVIAN MODEL APPLIED TO PLANNING
FOR CARDIOVASCULAR DISEASES

This example deals with the application of the model described above to the planning of personal health services for patients with cardiovascular diseases (390–458 in *International Classification of Diseases*, World Health Organization, Health Statistics, Eighth Revision) at the levels of primary medical care, consultant medical care, community hospital and teaching hospital care for a hypothetical region with a population of two million people that is increasing at an annual rate of 1·2 per cent.

The 'population not utilizing medical or hospital care' in this example includes that fraction of the total population not under medical or hospital care associated with cardiovascular diseases. It includes people with untreated cardiovascular diseases as well as those without these conditions. The primary medical care, consultant medical care, community hospital and teaching hospital care states include people receiving each of these levels of care because they have a diagnosed cardiovascular disease.

Prediction

The following two tables illustrate the inputs for the prediction model.

TABLE 12

INPUTS IN THE PREDICTION MODEL (I)

Empirical estimates of the transitional probabilities.

		STATE OF MEDICAL AND HOSPITAL CARE				
i STATE \ *j* STATE \ STATE OF MEDICAL AND HOSPITAL CARE		*Population not utilizing medical or hospital care*	*Primary medical care*	*Consultant medical care*	*Community hospital care*	*Teaching hospital care*
		1	2	3	4	5
Population not utilizing medical or hospital care	1	0·923	0·035	0·004	0	0
Primary medical care .	2	0·324	0·552	0·076	0·044	0·008
Consultant medical care .	3	0·528	0·242	0·182	0·008	0·032
Community hospital care	4	0·073	0·054	0·054	0·800	0·016
Teaching hospital care .	5	0·115	0·077	0·098	0·044	0·662

TABLE 12 presents empirical estimates of the transitional probabilities, representing all possible flows among the health services states in this numerical example. Empirical transitional probabilities are those calculated during the empirical time period, that is, the unit of time over which the number of people transiting from state i to state j has been calculated. If the empirical time periods were the same for all transitional probabilities, then the sum of those in the same row would add up to one.

In this table, the referrals from primary and consultant medical care are the transitional probabilities for three-month periods, while those from community and teaching hospital care are daily transitional probabilities. The data on flow from the 'population not utilizing medical or hospital care' are annual transitional probabilities. The use of different empirical time periods reflects the difficulty of obtaining adequate data, but does not impair the logic supporting the model.

TABLE 13

INPUTS IN THE PREDICTION MODEL (II)

Initial fractions $Pi(O)$, at state i, for cardiovascular diseases.

STATE OF MEDICAL AND HOSPITAL CARE (i)	Population not utilizing medical or hospital care	Primary medical care	Consultant medical care	Com-munity hospital care	Teaching hospital care
	1	2	3	4	5
$P_i(O)$	0·9621	0·0273	0·0037	0·0043	0·0008

TABLE 13 illustrates the empirical estimates of the initial fractions of the total population in each of the health services states. The empirical estimates presented in this numerical example have been adapted from different sources (White and Ibrahim, 1963; *Scottish Hospital In-Patient Statistics, 1965*, Table 7; *Report on the Hospital In-Patient Enquiry for the year 1960*, Part II, Table 13; Densen, Balamuth, and Deardorff, 1960). The data is merely illustrative and no significance should be attached to the particular numbers used.

The outputs of the model are those fractions of the population in the different health services states that are calculated to be present at different time periods. If these fractions are known, the required manpower and facility resources for the total population can be calculated.

The unbroken lines in FIGURE 25 show the predicted number of physicians in primary and consultant medical care required for the exclusive care of cardiovascular conditions in the above-mentioned population. In FIGURE 26 the unbroken lines show the predicted number of community and teaching hospital beds required for the exclusive care of cardiovascular conditions in the same population.

Simulation

Simulation consists of studying the repercussions that changes in the system, associated with changes in the transitional probability matrix, have on utilization of health services, and the consequent requirements in resources at different time periods.

For example, suppose that, as a result of a proposed mass screening programme for cardiovascular diseases, the number of persons with these diseases entering the primary medical care state during one year doubled and

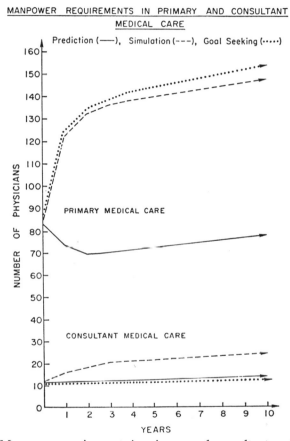

MANPOWER REQUIREMENTS IN PRIMARY AND CONSULTANT MEDICAL CARE

Prediction (——), Simulation (---), Goal Seeking (·····)

FIG. 25. Manpower requirements in primary and consultant medical care.

the number referred for consultant medical care increased by a quarter; since the health services system is regarded as an interdependent whole rather than as the sum of its independent states, an administrator responsible for the health of the population in this region might ask for an estimate of the repercussions this change would have on the utilization of the various health services and on their resource requirements.

The situation is simulated in the Markovian model by multiplying the transitional probability of a patient with cardiovascular disease going from state 'population not utilizing medical or hospital care' to state 'primary medical care' by two, and the transitional probability from the state 'population not utilizing medical care and hospital care' to 'consultant medical care' by five-fourths.

The output of the simulation model in this application is the estimated utilization indicated by the new fractions of the population in each health services state at different time periods. This new set of fractions will determine the new set of requirements.

The broken lines in FIGURE 25 reflect the new manpower required as a result of the simulated situation, while those in FIGURE 26 reflect the new facility requirements in the simulated situation.

The simulated mass screening for cardiovascular diseases mentioned above in the population of two million people would require, for instance, at the end of five years the following additional manpower and facility resources for the exclusive care of patients with those conditions:

1. 68 more primary care physicians.
2. 8 more specialists or consultants.
3. 976 more community hospital beds.
4. 172 more teaching hospital beds.

Goal-seeking

Goal-seeking aims to determine that alternative which will minimize a given constraint in order to reach a specified goal.

In the health services system described, planning services for the care of patients with cardiovascular diseases in the hypothetical region with two million people might include the goal of doubling in ten years the number of patients with cardiovascular diseases under primary medical care, while utilization of other levels of care remained the same. It might also include the knowledge that there will be few additional resources available at that time. The health services administrator might ask how current resources should be utilized, at different time periods, to reach the desired objective in such a way that minimal additional resources are required. In other words, the problem is to choose the utilization strategy that will minimize change in current resources to reach the specified goal.

In goal-seeking the input to the model is current utilization (defined by current fractions of the population in each state), desired utilization during the time designated, and the utilization parameters. A further input is the constraint that must be minimized by the alternative chosen.

The output of the model would be the optimum utilization strategy, at different time periods, that will reach the specified goal with minimum change in current resources.

The dotted line in FIGURE 25 shows the calculated number of primary and consultant medical care physicians required, at different time periods, in order to meet the goal presented in the goal-seeking model. In FIGURE 26, the

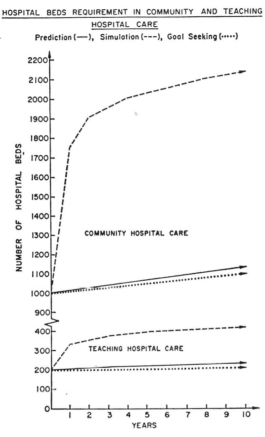

FIG. 26. Hospital beds requirement in community and teaching hospital care.

dotted line shows the number of community and teaching hospital beds required at different periods, to meet the given goal.

Other Applications

This Markovian model can be expanded to include two new states, birth and death, and different transitional probabilities matrices for each age group. It thus enables one to consider the different utilization rates of personal health services by different age groups. With this expansion, the model takes into account first, changes in size and age structure of the population, and secondly, the different utilization experiences of the different age groups (Navarro, 1968).

APPENDIX 1

ESTIMATING THE PROBABILITY OF GOING FROM HEALTH SERVICES STATE i TO STATE j DURING THE FUNDAMENTAL TIME INTERVAL

P_{ij}, the transitional probability, denotes the probability that a person in state i at the beginning of the empirical time period will go to state j during that period. The empirical time period, T_{ij}, is the unit of time over which the number of people, n_{ij} (T_{ij}), have moved from state i to state j.

$$P_{ij} = \frac{n_{ij}\,(T_{ij})}{n_i} \tag{1}$$

The transitional probability, P_{ij}, given for different empirical time periods, T_{ij}, is translated into daily transitional probabilities, i.e. the time period of one day is selected as the fundamental one because this is the period of time during which it is highly unlikely that a person will be in more than one state. Thus, any duplication in calculating the number of persons in each of the different states is avoided. The fundamental time period is that chosen to define the transitional probability matrix. In this matrix, the sum of all elements in the same row add up to one.

The daily transitional probabilities are obtained from

$$q_{ij} = \frac{P_{ij}\,(T_{ij})}{T_{ij}}, \quad i \neq j \tag{2}$$

where: q_{ij} is the probability of going from state i to state j during a fundamental time interval of one day.

$P_{ij}(T_{ij})$ is the probability of going from state i to state j during the empirical time period T_{ij}.

T_{ij} is the empirical time period in days.

The daily transitional probability matrix, Q, is defined by

$$Q = \begin{pmatrix} q_{11} & q_{12} & \cdots & q_{1k} \\ q_{21} & q_{22} & \cdots & q_{2k}, \\ & \cdots & & \\ q_{k1} & q_{k2} & \cdots & q_{kk} \end{pmatrix}$$

where k is the number of states.

APPENDIX 2

CALCULATING RESOURCES REQUIREMENTS

Knowing the health services state fractions $P_i(t)$, the manpower ($MD =$ physicians) and facilities ($BEDS$) requirements are calculated from formulas (3) and (4).

$$R_{MD_i}(t) = \frac{\dfrac{P_i(t)\,N(t)}{L_i} \times \gamma_i \times 365}{\theta_i} \tag{3}$$

where: $R_{MD_i}(t)$ is the number of physicians for state i (as a function of time t).

$P_i(t)$ is the fraction in state i at time t.

$N(t)$ is the size of population base, at time t, and determined by the rate of population growth.

L_i is the average length of stay in health services state i and is equal to the fraction $q_{ii}/(1\text{-}q_{ii})$, (q_{ii}, daily probability of remaining in state i).

γ_i is the number of visits per entry at state i.

$\dfrac{P_i(t)\,N(t)}{L_i}$ is the number of entries to state i per day.

It may help to clarify this formula if $P_i(t)\ N(t)$ is considered to be prevalence. Prevalence is then equal to the number of entries, i.e. incidence, per day, multiplied by the average length of stay.

Altogether, the numerator $P_i(t)\ N(t) \times \gamma_i \times 365/L_i$ is the number of visits required for state i per year. θ_i, the denominator, is the average physician load factor or the number of visits at state i per physician per year.

Similarly, the requirements for beds is calculated with formula (4).

$$R_{BEDS}(t) = \frac{P_i(t)\,N(t)}{F_i} \tag{4}$$

where F_i is the occupancy desired at state i.

APPENDIX 3

CALCULATING $P_i(t)$: FRACTIONS OF THE TOTAL POPULATION IN HEALTH SERVICES STATE i, AT TIME PERIOD t.

The predicted fractions of the population (or probabilities of being in the states) in time period t is given by the expression (5).

$$\overrightarrow{P(t)} = \overrightarrow{P(O)}\ Q^t \tag{5}$$

where: $\overrightarrow{P(t)}$ is the vector representing the fractions of the population in the
                different states, at time t days.
$\overrightarrow{P(O)}$ is the vector representing the initial fractions of the population
                in the different states.
Q is the daily transitional probability matrix.
t is the time in days from the initial period to the end of the t
                time period.

Thus, given $P_i\ (O)$ and P_{ij}, one may predict $P_i\ (t)$ using the Markovian assumptions.

In simulation, the same mathematical model is used.

In goal-seeking, the solution of the problem is to minimize 'the amount of change' subject to reaching the desired goal. This minimizing change is embodied in the selection of the objective function in a mathematical quadratic program.[1] The problem solved is:

$$\underset{\{P^1_{ij}\}}{\text{minimize}} \sum_{i}^{k}\sum_{j}^{k} W_{ij}(P^1_{ij} - P_{ij})^2 \qquad (6)$$
$$\text{subject to } \overrightarrow{P(\infty)} = \overrightarrow{P(\infty)} \cdot Q^1.$$

The objective function is the weighted Euclidian distance between the solution 'referral rates' P^1_{ij} and the current referral rates, P_{ij}. The problem then is to minimize the change of referral pattern necessary to effect a desired steady state vector $\overrightarrow{P(\infty)}$ of fractions of the population in the various health services states.[2]

The terms 'constraint' and 'limitation' have been used in some instances in place of 'objective function', for purposes of comprehensibility to the non-mathematical reader. It is hoped that this flexibility of notation will not cause any confusion.

REFERENCES

AHUMADA, J., GUZMAN, A. A., DURAN, H., PIZZI, M., SARUE, E., and TESTA, M. (1965) *Health Planning: Problems of Concept and Method*, Pan American Health Organization, Publication No. III, Washington D.C.

ANDERSON, T. W. (1954) Probability models for analysing time changes in attitudes in *Mathematical Thinking in the Social Sciences*, ed. Lazarsfeld, P. F., Glencoe, Ill.

BAILEY, N. T. J. (1967) *The Mathematical Approach to Biology and Medicine*, New York.

BARTHOLOMEW, D. T. (1967) *Stochastic Models for Social Processes*, New York.

[1] The quadratic program used in goal-seeking has been programmed for the computer by Judith Liebman under P.H.S. Grant HM (00279).

[2] For a mathematical description of quadratic programming see Navarro and Parker (1967). For a broad description of mathematical programming see Garvin (1960).

BLUMEN, I., KOGAN, M., and MCCARTHY, P. T. (1955) *The Industrial Mobility of Labour as a Probability Process*, Cornell Studies in Industrial and Labour Relations, Ithaca, N.Y.

BUSH, R. R., and MOSTELLER, F. (1955) *Stochastic Models for Learning*, New York.

DENSON, P. M., BALAMUTH, E., and DEARDORFF, N. R. (1960) Medical care plans as a source of morbidity data, *Milbank mem. Fd Quart.*, **38**, 101.

DIVISION OF INDIAN HEALTH (1966) *Program Packaging*, United States Public Health Services, Washington, D.C.

DOOB, J. L. (1962) *Stochastic Processes*, New York.

ESTES, W. K. (1950) Towards a statistical theory of learning, *Psychol. Rev.*, **57**, 94.

FELLER, W. (1957) *An Introduction to the Probability Theory and its Applications*, New York.

FIX, E., and NEYMAN, J. (1951) A simple stochastic model of recovery, relapse, death and loss of patients, *Hum. Biol.*, **23**, 205.

FLAGLE, C. D., HUGGINS, W. H., and ROY, R. H. (1960) *Operations Research and Systems Engineering*, Baltimore, Md.

GARVIN, W. W. (1960) *Introduction to Linear Programming*, New York.

HARARY, F., and LIPSTEIN, B. (1962) The dynamics of brand loyalty: a Markovian approach, *Operations Research*, **10**, 19.

HOPE, K., and SKRIMSHIRE, A. (1968) *Patients Flows in the National Health Services: A Markov Analysis*, Health Services Research and Intelligence Unit, Scottish Home and Health Department (processed), Edinburgh.

KEMENY, T. G., and SNELL, J. L. (1960) *Finite Markov Chains*, Princeton, N.J.

KLARMAN, H. E., FRANCIS, J. O., and ROSENTHAL, G. D. (1968) Cost effectiveness analysis applied to the treatment of chronic renal disease, *Med. Care*, **6**, 48.

LAST, J. (1963) The iceberg—completing the clinical picture—in general practice, *Lancet*, ii, 28.

MARSHALL, A. N., and GOLDHAMMER, H. (1955) An application of Markov processes to the study of the epidemiology of mental disease, *J. Amer. statist. Ass.*, **50**, 99.

MINISTRY OF HEALTH AND GENERAL REGISTER OFFICE (1963) *Report on Hospital In-Patient Inquiry for the Year 1960*, Part II, detailed tables, London, H.M.S.O., Table 13, p. 156.

NAVARRO, V. (1968) *Planning Personal Health Services: A Markovian Model*, Dr.P.H. Dissertation, Department of Medical Care and Hospitals, Johns Hopkins University, Baltimore, Md.

NAVARRO, V. (1969) Systems approach to health planning, *Hlth Serv. Res.*, **4**, 96.

NAVARRO, V. (1970) A review of methods used in planning the distribution of personal health services, in *Survey of Health Planning*, ed. Reinke, W. A., Baltimore, Md.

NAVARRO, V., and PARKER, R. D. (1967) *A Planning Model for Personal Health Services*, Department of Medical Care and Hospitals, Johns Hopkins University, Baltimore, Md.

NAVARRO, V., and PARKER, R. D. (1968) A mathematical model for health planning: prediction, simulation and goal-seeking, *Proceedings of the Fifth Scientific Meeting of the International Epidemiological Association, Primosten, Yugoslavia.*

PRAIS, S. F. (1955) Measuring social mobility, *J. roy. statist. Soc.*, **118**, 56.

REINKE, W. A. (1970) *Quantitative Decision Procedures*, Baltimore, Md.

SCOTTISH HOME AND HEALTH DEPARTMENT (1967) *Scottish Hospital In-Patient Statistics, 1965*, Edinburgh, Table 7, p. 48.

SINGER, S. (1961) *A Stochastic Model of Variation of Categories of Patients within a Hospital*, Ph.D. Dissertation, School of Engineering, Johns Hopkins University, Baltimore, Md.

SVERDRUP, E. (1965) Estimates and test procedures in connection with stochastic models of deaths, recoveries, and transfers between different states of health, *Skand Aktuar*, **46**, 184.

WHITE, K. L. (1967) Improved medical care statistics and the health services system, *Publ. Hlth Rep. (Wash.)*, **82**, 847.

WHITE, K. L., and IBRAHIM, M. A. (1963) The distribution of cardiovascular disease in the community, *Ann. intern. Med.*, **56**, 631.

ZAHL, S. (1955) A Markov process model for follow-up studies, *Hum. Biol.*, **27**, 90.

PART VII

IMPLICATIONS

15

IMPLICATIONS OF FINDINGS FOR HEALTH POLICY

LESTER BRESLOW

HEALTH policy on a world scale or in a nation is determined by many factors, including the nature of health problems, technology available to cope with them, resources that can potentially be allocated to health programmes, and social forces expressed in the competition for available resources.

Findings derived from the application of epidemiological techniques are becoming increasingly important elements in determining health policy. Epidemiology not only delineates health problems and elucidates the factors responsible for them but can also be used to guide efforts to deal with the problems. Understanding gained through epidemiology has become a major means of directing large-scale efforts to control diseases that once devastated mankind. For example, the concept, procedures, and guide-lines for the campaigns for global control of smallpox and malaria are derived in large part from epidemiological studies.

DELINEATING APPROACHES TO HEALTH PROBLEMS

Recently improved methods of data handling enhance the ability of epidemiology to strengthen programmes designed to control health problems. Where there is a choice of method for control, epidemiological studies can indicate which approaches are most promising, and health advances will increasingly be based upon clarification of the three major ways of attacking health problems:

1. Environmental health measures.
2. Medical care.
3. Health education.

They will also be based upon determination of which one or which combination of these is most useful for particular problems.

Take, for example, automobile accidents—a health problem of growing magnitude throughout the world that calls for use of all three of the above approaches.

Environmental

Defects in the design of automobiles are now recognized as an important factor in the injuries and fatalities associated with automobile accidents. In the United States and other countries, manufacturers, stimulated by epidemiological data showing that the physical construction of automobiles plays a role in accidental injuries and death, are incorporating specific safety features into automobiles in order to minimize the occurrence and reduce the impact of accidents. Furthermore, recognition of faults in the steering mechanism and other components of automobiles after their production, sale, and use by thousands of drivers is leading to factory recall of large numbers of vehicles for correction of the defects (Fisher, 1965).

Another significant environmental aspect of automobile accidents, of course, is the design of roadways. Identification of stretches of road which involve a high risk of accident, followed by detailed engineering studies of such situations, leads both to corrective action and better planning of future roadways.

Medical Care

Even after accidents occur, emergency medical services based upon modern techniques can minimize deaths and reduce disability resulting from them. Appropriate distribution of such medical services in rural and urban areas can be guided by epidemiological study (Waller, Garner, and Lawrence, 1966). The latter can thus contribute not only to understanding the factors that determine the occurrence of disease, including accidents, but also to understanding the factors that determine the outcome of injuries. Among these medical care is increasingly important; health policy must include both prevention and treatment. Epidemiology can aid both.

Health Education

The personal, or driver, factor in automobile accidents has long been known to be important, especially the impairment of driving ability associated with alcohol consumption. For many years, however, attention focused on the so-called 'social drinker' who took one drink too many before getting behind the wheel. While this type of drinking is not insignificant, epidemiological studies have shown that fatalities from automobile accidents are highly concentrated among heavy drinkers (McCarroll and Haddon, 1962). Programmes designed to reduce deaths from automobile accidents through changing behaviour, that is, through health education, must take into account the nature of drinking involved and the identification of individuals with the greatest risk. Efforts should be concentrated on habitual heavy drinkers.

Considering the magnitude and complexity of the health problem involved in automobile accidents, new methods of data handling for epidemiological investigation may be extremely valuable in developing health policy. Large-scale information systems for registration of drivers and automobiles, recording of accidents and the circumstances in which they occur, record linkage of such data to types of vehicles, roadways, and persons (for example, known alcoholics), and systematic use of such information systems, could greatly enhance efforts to control this important health hazard.

Identification of circumstances and persons with a high risk for automobile accidents is now just as feasible as it was for typhoid fever in the past. Such identification, however, depends to a considerable degree on the proper use of large-scale information systems. Based on these systems, the application of epidemiology to the problem of automobile accidents carries as much promise for guiding health policy as it formerly did for typhoid fever.

AUTOMATED MULTIPHASIC SCREENING

One may examine the implication of modern methods of data handling not only from the standpoint of a particular health problem, such as automobile accidents, but also from that of a particular technique which can contribute to the solution of several health problems, for example, automated multiphasic screening.

Multiphasic screening consists of a battery of tests and examinations for the presumptive identification of diseases in persons not known to have them. Tuberculosis, diabetes, cancer of the cervix, and many other important conditions can be detected in individuals who present no symptoms or other indication of such serious disease. Screening by itself is, of course, not diagnostic; it must be followed by referral of the patient together with the results of screening to a physician for definitive diagnosis and any necessary therapy.

Automated multiphasic screening incorporates into the process the automation of several laboratory tests and computerized data processing. For example, Collen has described one automated multiphasic screening laboratory as including electrocardiogram, chest X-ray, mammography, anthropometry, blood pressure, visual acuity, tonometry, respirometry, ankle test, hearing, medical questionnaire and laboratory determinations of haemoglobin, white cell count, serological test for syphilis, rheumatoid factor, blood grouping, eight serum chemistry determinations (glucose, creatinine, albumin, total protein, cholesterol, uric acid, calcium and transaminase), and urine tests for pH, blood, glucose, protein, and bacteria. The entire periodic health evaluation includes these procedures, plus a physical examination performed at a subsequent appointment by an internist, and supplemental examinations such as cervical smear for cancer detection. Computerized processing of the multiphasic screening data yields 'on line', before the individual has left the laboratory, 'advice as to any additional procedure which it would be advisable for the patient to receive in order to assist in achieving a more specific diagnosis. These "advice" rules have been previously established by the internists, and instruct the receptionist to arrange certain additional tests and appointments for the patient before his physical examination visit with the physician'. Computer collation of all data, including that received after the laboratory visit (such as interpretation of the X-ray), yields 'off-line' comparison of findings with certain predetermined 'consider' rules in the form of suggestions to the physician that he 'consider' certain diagnostic categories. The physician reviews the report at the time of the patient's visit and takes further steps to arrive at final diagnosis (Collen, 1967).

Detection of Disease

Automated multiphasic screening carries many implications for health policy. It offers, first of all, the opportunity to detect many cases of disease in their early stages when the outlook for treatment is presumably most favourable. Furthermore, it does this with an economical unit–cost per test. Collen estimates that 'to provide this same battery of tests by traditional non-automated methods would cost four to five times as much' (Collen *et al.*, 1969). Savings in health manpower are obvious.

Even more significant from the epidemiological standpoint, when applied repeatedly to tens of thousands of persons over a period of several years, automated multiphasic screening and diagnostic follow-up by physicians can yield more complete knowledge than was available in the past about the distribution of disease in populations. It is a systematic means of obtaining such information about large populations, superior to relying upon physicians reporting cases that come to attention in the usual manner. The latter, largely dependent upon patient-recognition of symptoms and subsequent physician-diagnosis, includes only a fraction of the cases that actually exist and can be disclosed through automated multiphasic screening. More precise knowledge about the occurrence of disease in various segments of the population is obviously an advantage in guiding health services.

Understanding Disease Processes

Automated multiphasic screening also opens up the possibility of learning more about the natural history of several significant conditions. For example, the progression of the condition characterized only by slightly increased blood pressure into hypertension and hypertensive heart disease, or of slightly impaired glucose tolerance into diabetes, or slightly elevated ocular tension into glaucoma—such aspects of disease are poorly understood at present. The pattern of progression, that is, how rapidly and under what circumstances this progression occurs, as well as the proportion of persons in whom progression occurs after the early signs mentioned above, can be ascertained by large-scale follow-up of individuals in whom abnormalities are detected.

If large groups of people are subjected to automated multiphasic screening and if definite, though arbitrary, limits of 'abnormal' response to tests are established as the basis for treatment of various diseases, there also arises the possibility of a more rational approach to treatment of early disease. Collen and his group have initiated a series of so-called 'spin-off' studies, for example, on hypertension. Clinicians hold varying opinions as to whether moderately high blood pressure, with no other evidence of disease, should be practically ignored, treated mildly with drugs, or treated aggressively with drugs. With such difference of opinion and lack of evidence as to what constitutes the best course, automated multiphasic screening of large groups of people creates an opportunity for therapeutic trials. While these involve clinical rather than epidemiological skills, automated multiphasic screening does bring the clinician and the epidemiologist together at an important point for the understanding of disease—namely, the identification of persons with 'abnormal' tests, but not frank clinical disease, and what happens to them.

Another example of spin-off studies is the evaluation of treating asymptomatic patients with impaired carbohydrate tolerance by means of oral hypoglycaemic drugs, in order to determine their effectiveness in preventing overt diabetes (Collen, 1967).

Revolutionizing Health Services

The major implication of automated multiphasic screening for health policy emerges from the possibility that such studies may show an advantage in detecting and treating physiological and anatomical abnormalities before disease in its usual form can be recognized. If this proves true for several conditions, the implication for health policy would be enormous. It would probably, in fact, revolutionize our whole approach to health services for those chronic diseases in which physiological and anatomical abnormalities appear before frank disease can be recognized. The diseases of the latter half of the twentieth century, particularly the most important ones, seem to be mainly of this type. Thus, if the presumption about early detection and aggressive treatment of such conditions proves true, our whole approach to such diseases would have to change. Instead of waiting for individuals to come to the physician with symptoms, the health services would have to be organized to bring in individuals for periodic assessment through automated multiphasic screening and appropriate follow-up. One of the principal concerns of the health services would then be the physiological surveillance of the entire population and the appropriate treatment of abnormalities discovered, before frank disease could be recognized either by the patient or physician.

It is now rare to find individuals in diabetic coma where people have access to excellent medical services. A condition which was common only a few decades ago has become uncommon because scientific and technological advance has led to improved medical service. If automated multiphasic screening demonstrates its effectiveness as a means of reducing morbidity and mortality from diabetes and other chronic diseases investigated in the long-term studies now under way, health services will have to be vastly reorganized.

Instead of being geared to treatment of frank clinical entities, they should be aimed at detecting abnormal conditions in their early stages, through participation of the population in automated multiphasic screening, and at follow-up treatment. Prevention should become an integral part of health care.

Thus, we see that automated multiphasic screening carries the potential of revolutionizing health services. To guide the rigorous evaluation of the process, epidemiologic studies involving large-scale data handling are clearly necessary.

REFERENCES

COLLEN, M. F. (1967) Computer analyses in preventive health research, *Meth. Inform. Med.*, **6**, 1.

COLLEN, M. F. (1968) Automated multiphasic screening, in *Presymptomatic Detection and Early Diagnosis*, ed. Sharp, C. L., Baltimore, Md., p. 65.

COLLEN, M. F. *et al.* (1969) Cost analysis of a multiphasic screening program, *New Engl. J. Med.*, **280**, 1043.

FISHER, P. (1965) Dangerously designed automobiles, *Northw. Med.* (*Seattle*), **64(6)**, 417.

McCARROLL, J., and HADDON, W., JNR. (1962) A controlled study of fatal automobile accidents in New York City, *J. chron. Dis.*, **15**, 811.

WALLER, J. A., GARNER, R., and LAWRENCE, R. (1966) Utilisation of ambulance services in a rural community, *Publ. Hlth* (*Lond.*), **56(3)**, 513.

INDEX

INDEX

Analysis and computers, 3, 124–9
—, canonical variate, 149, 155–61
—, cluster, 7, 149, 161–6
—, component, 125, 163
—, discriminant, 8, 149, 155–6
—, dispersion, 163–4
—, multivariate, 6, 31, 149–66
— of covariance, 125
— of survey data, 5, 8–10
— of variance, 125, 150, 152
—, profile, 149, 150–5, 164–5
—, regression, 8, 9, 125, 187
Asthma, 5
Atmospheric pollution, 18, 28

Behavioural patterns and health, 25, 35–7

Cancer, follow-up of patients, 65, 88, 90, 104, 184
— of cervix, 203
— of lung, 30, 35, 47, 86
— of stomach, 29
Cardiovascular diseases, 181, 189, 190, 191, 192
Case-control studies, *see* Retrospective studies
Cholera, 21, 63
Chronic bronchitis, 29, 45, 46, 47, 48–9, 50–1, 74
Chronic disease and screening, 28–9, 205–6
— — and virus infection, 18, 29
— —, prevention of, 6, 35–7
— —, registration of, 64
Classification of psychiatric patients, 150–2, 161–6
Clusters of conditions, 7, 29
Cohort studies, 6, 31
Communicable disease, 14, 15–26
— — and environmental conditions, 18, 23
— — control, 16, 20–3, 25, 201
— — eradication, 20, 23, 25, 141–2
— — investigation of outbreaks of, 24–5
— — notification of, 16, 63–4
— — prevention of, 16, 33–5
— — transmission or spread of, 15, 17–20, 21
Computers and classification of psychiatric patients, 162–3, 164–6
— and drug usage, 39–40

— and epidemiology, 3, 14, 31–2, 124–32
— and identification, 99, 101
— and medical records, 41, 67, 84, 92, 104, 106–7
— and multiple causes of death, 62
— and record linkage, 67, 83–4, 92–3, 99, 104, 107
— and screening, 203–5
— and survey analysis, 8, 47, 111, 118–22
— and survey planning, 126
— and teaching, 131–2
Congenital disease, 14, 37, 89
Controlled trials of vaccines, 33–4
— — of patient care, 6, 39, 40, 88, 205
Cost-benefit analysis and medical care, 183
Cross-sectional studies, *see* Prevalence studies

Data banks, 106, 129, 130–1
— 'dredging', 8, 126
—, editing of, 3, 9–10
— formats, 124–5
— processing, 3, 112, 115, 118–22, 125
— recording, 112–16
— 'reduction', 169
—, retrieval of, 66, 67, 94, 130
—, routine collection of, 55–67
—, storage of, 66, 67, 118–19, 130–1
—, tabulation of, 5, 121–2, 125
Death certification, 60–2, 83, 84, 89, 103
Developing countries, communicable disease in, 25
— —, identification in, 94–101
Diabetes, 203, 204, 205
Diphtheria, 20, 22, 64, 91
Drugs, monitoring of, 37, 66, 131
—, resistance to, 17
—, trials of, 33–5
—, usage of, 39–40

Effectiveness and medical care, 40, 183
Efficiency and medical care, 183
Enumeration, 112, 113–15
—, errors in, 57
Epidemics and mathematical models, 7–8, 129–30, 135–47
—, prediction of, 17, 18, 19, 131
—, prevention of, 18